CW01096003

Tired of Feeling Tired?

Tina Christoudias-Spyrou,
MBA, RDN

Clinical Dietitian, Nutritionist

Cover design: Ioanna Pattichi

Edited by: Sandra J. Judd

Disclaimer

The medical information in this book is provided as an educational resource only, and is not intended to be used or relied upon for any diagnostic or treatment purposes. This information should not be used as a substitute for professional diagnosis and treatment.

The nutritional interventions discussed in this book should not be used as a substitute for conventional medical therapy.

Furthermore, none of the statements in this book have been evaluated by the Food and Drug Administration.

Please consult your health-care provider before making any health-care decisions or for guidance about a specific medical condition.

Dedication

I dedicate this book to all those who suffer from hypothyroidism as well as those who have found the strength to take their health into their own hands.

.

TIRED OF FEELING TIRED?

TABLE OF CONTENTS

Acknowledgements

I would like to thank my parents, John and Aphrodite, who taught me that life belongs to those who dare. Without them, I would not have the courage and the strength to fight for what I believe in. Thanks Mom and Dad for instilling such high values and standards in me.

I would also like to thank my husband, Spyros, for the unrelenting love and support he continues to give me on this journey of life we are on together. The sacrifices he made while I was writing this book and on my journey to healing can never be repaid. I am grateful for such an amazing partner.

I thank my children Aphrodite, Demetris, and Stefanos for being my cheerleaders no matter what and for keeping my spirits high.

I would also like to thank my brother, Mario, who is an inspiration to me because of his strong work ethic, his contagious personality, and his consistently positive attitude. His friendship has been invaluable to me.

It goes without saying that many thanks also go out to my smart, passionate, and visionary colleagues, Vanessa and Christina, who inspire me to pursue higher levels of knowledge and success on a daily basis.

MY STORY

I am a recovering victim of hypothyroidism. Why do I call myself a victim? Well, let me tell you a story to give you a better picture.

In my twenties, I was a person who was full of life. I loved to be outdoors, I listened to all types of music, I sang opera, I had an active social life, and I spent a lot of time reading and studying. Anyone who has ever known me will tell you how silly and full of smiles I was. In my thirties, however, things drastically changed. I found myself tired all the time. I couldn't concentrate or focus, I slept for hours, gained weight, lost a lot of hair, had constipation, and was depressed. I suspected that I had a thyroid problem, as I had lived through my mother having thyroid disease. Unfortunately, I was right.

The up-beat and fun-loving spirit that everyone knew was no more. I seldom smiled and could not muster up the energy to even go for a walk outside. So, I did what everyone does when they do not feel well. I went to the doctor.

"Oh my God!" the doctor said. "You have one of the highest TSH levels I have ever seen. Ok, the answer is clear here. Let's start you on thyroxine." A glimmer of hope. I would start taking these magic pills and finally start to feel better!

Unfortunately, that day never came. I continued to feel low and exhausted. I would spend my days sitting on the couch for hours with only enough energy to walk back and forth to the kitchen. What did I do to make myself feel some sort of comfort? Eat all the foods that I was not supposed to. Mainly foods made up of white flour and sugar.

Now, one would think that the above scenario would be unthinkable for a trained, registered dietitian such as myself. After all, I had all the tools I needed to take care of myself. I had the power to heal myself, right? Wrong! In our training, we are not taught how nutrition can heal the body. We are taught how it can maintain a desperate disease state. Our professors talked about diabetes *maintenance* or weight *maintenance*. We seldom heard about how nutrition could be the game changer when faced with a chronic ailment.

After seeing me suffer for so long, my husband gave me something that changed my life. He went on the internet and found a book called, *Stop the Thyroid Madness*. Thank you Janie A. Bowthorpe for opening my eyes. Ms. Bowthorpe is not a nutrition professional but she is a person who wanted answers, as I did. From that book, I discovered that thyroxine-only therapy was doing nothing for me and that there were better alternatives.

To make a long story short, I found a doctor of integrative medicine, Dr. David Owen, while on holiday in England. I owe a lot to this man as he started me on the journey toward recovery. He gave me nutritional supplements and gave me some pointers on how to change my diet (no irony there!). After only one week of making a few changes, my brain fog lifted (and my intestines began to function! Yay!).

Well, this was only the beginning of the journey for me. Using my scientific background and my knowledge in nutrition to my advantage, I started to look for more answers. I discovered that eating organic, natural foods and avoiding grains and all processed foods really put me on the road to recovery. The answer had been in my hands all along. The secret to recovery was in nature and in my food. I started to explore holistic nutrition and functional medicine tactics and with my clinical background, I started to put the pieces of the thyroid puzzle together.

So, why was I a victim? I was a victim because the medical community, the way I was trained as a nutritionist, and the food industry failed me. I am not saying that doctors and my education are useless. I am saying that I discovered that we as a global community, put unyielding trust in a system that falls short of treating chronic disease.

What do I mean? We eat foods prepared by fast-food companies and restaurants because it just looks and smells so good. We use toxic substances to clean our homes. We barely go outside to connect with nature. We pop pills to make our headaches go away instead of exploring why the headaches are happening in the first place. We buy our children sugar- laden cereal, believing that we are giving them something healthy. We are money obsessed and therefore stressed out to no end. Doesn't this sound like an equation for disease? Of course it does! Our bodies, minds, and spirits all need balance to exist happily and peacefully. The answer to treating your thyroid problem is not just in a pill, but in completely altering your lifestyle from your psychology to the type of water you drink.

I wrote this book in order to share my personal experience and scientific expertise with those who suffer from thyroid disease. I feel where all of you are coming from, because I, too, was in a dark place for a long time. I wrote this book as a living testament to how a holistic lifestyle with real food *can* heal you and *can* bring you to the healthy person you want to be. I hope this small contribution will help change lives and inspire people to spread the word about holistic therapy. I wish you a happy journey to good health!

As the issue of hypothyroidism is complex, the focus of this book will be on research that supports nutrition protocols for supporting thyroid treatment. Nutrition therapy is a game changer for many chronic diseases and should definitely be employed when trying to improve health and overall quality of life. It is beyond the scope of this book to discuss in detail laboratory and other tests, medications, and other issues with which only a doctor or functional medicine practitioner can help you.

My Personal Experience with Hypothyroidism

After feeling tired and run-down for so long, I was relieved to find out that I could take thyroxine and start to feel better. When that did not happen and I really explored more about the disease, as with many other diseases like cardiovascular disease and cancer, I found that hypothyroidism is the culmination of a variety of different factors and that it takes years to develop.

Sure, we can blame this on genes, but research shows that we have control over which genes are turned on and which genes stay dormant. The particular study of genetics that I talk about is called epigenetics. There is even a sub-section of this area of study called nutri-epigenetics. Nutri-epigenetics looks at how food can turn genes on or off.

Epigenetics and the role of how food affects gene regulation are too involved to get into. I recommend you read my colleague Christina Economidou's book, *Anti-Cancer, The Preventive Power of Food*, for a great example of how nutrition can change our genes to protect against cancer.

The reason I brought up epigenetics at all is that, like other diseases, hypothyroidism can be prevented as well as put into remission by diet. The thing I realized when looking for ways to heal myself was that hypothyroidism occurs because so many other things are going wrong in the body. The thyroid doesn't wake up one day and decide not to work. There are many factors that cause it to falter.

The adrenal glands, the intestines, the microbiome (the special blend of bacteria, viruses, and parasites that we all host), sex hormones, and the immune system all play a role in hypothyroidism. Therefore, all of these areas need to be addressed in order to heal. One can see why simply taking thyroxine without making necessary lifestyle changes falls short of decreasing hypothyroid symptoms.

The good news is that there are nutritional protocols that can be followed to address all of the afore-mentioned areas. Together with medication (or for some without), looking at the root cause of hypothyroidism and addressing it with nutrition can drastically change one's health outcome.

When I cut out foods like gluten and conventional dairy from my life, I literally started to feel better in a matter of days! My intestines worked better and I even saw the scale start to move in the right direction (for the first time in years). This dietary change, however, was only scratching the surface.

In this book, I talk about all of the areas that can contribute to hypothyroidism and I provide nutrition protocols that address each area. I present the research on foods that can boost thyroid function and discuss the foods that can hinder it. I also discuss other lifestyle factors, like stress, environmental toxins and chemicals, and exercise and how they can negatively or positively affect thyroid function.

Hypothyroidism is complicated. I drove myself crazy for many years trying to find answers to why I was feeling so low and depleted. Changing my diet, getting the right supplements, decreasing stress, and exercising all helped me to heal. My hope with this book is that you can find some nutrition solutions to help you on your journey to gaining health and feeling better.

CHAPTER 1

THYROID DISEASE BASICS

How the Thyroid Works

Let's start with the basics. The obvious way to better understand hypothyroidism is to look at the thyroid gland itself, how it functions, and how it affects the rest of the body.

The thyroid is a small butterfly-shaped organ found in the middle of the throat. As I have a music background, I like to refer to it as the conductor of the orchestra. It dictates how slow or fast, high or low, loud or soft, the music (in this case, the metabolic functioning of the body) will play.

The body needs thyroid hormones for the cells to produce energy, for the scalp to grow hair, for the intestines to digest food, for other hormones in the body to function properly, and for the brain to think. Without the right amount of thyroid hormones, the body, as an orchestra, is left to its own accord. Likewise, if some members of the orchestra (in this case the immune system, the gastro-intestinal tract, the adrenal glands, sex hormones, and the brain)start playing their own tune, thyroid function will also suffer. In other words, the thyroid needs the other systems in the body to function properly, just as the other systems in the body need the thyroid to do the same.

The thyroid is responsible for producing the hormones T4, T3, T2, T1, and calcitonin. To make things easy, however, we will focus on T4 and T3. T4 (thyroxine) is the stored form of thyroid hormone. In other words, it is not actively used by the cells to produce energy. T4 is converted to T3(triiodothyronine) which is the *active* form of thyroid hormone or the hormone that is used by the cells to produce energy.

When the thyroid produces a sufficient amount of both hormones, this creates a negative feedback loop, instructing the hypothalamus of the brain and the pituitary gland to tell the thyroid gland to continue to produce these hormones. However, when the thyroid produces either not enough or too much thyroid hormone, the hypothalamus and the pituitary gland instruct the thyroid to produce more or less hormone, respectively.

I wish the above explanation was good enough to make us fully comprehend the thyroid and how it works. It sounds easy, right? In the case of hypothyroidism, if you do not produce enough thyroid hormone, you simply need to supplement with extra (which in most cases, is with T4-only medication).

Unfortunately, the answer is that it is not necessarily that straightforward.

How common is hypothyroidism?

This is a tough question because it depends on a variety of things. Firstly, it depends on how a doctor would define hypothyroidism based on their interpretation of thyroid stimulating hormone (TSH) levels (the common blood test used to diagnose hypothyroidism). I say "interpretation" because experts today still cannot agree on what a normal or optimal range is for TSH. Knowing this fact and taking into consideration that many patients may not recognize the signs and symptoms of hypothyroidism, it becomes apparent that a lot of cases of a low-functioning thyroid may go unnoticed.

Adding to this confusion, hypothyroidism can also be classified into different categories: Hashimoto's thyroiditis (or autoimmune thyroiditis), hypothyroidism, and subclinical hypothyroidism. Therefore, depending on what parameters are being looked at, the prevalence of an underactive thyroid will vary.

In general, in countries that are iodine deficient, goiter formation and congenital hypothyroidism are seen. (A goiter is defined as the enlargement of the thyroid gland due to a deficiency in iodine). However, in countries such as the USA and Europe that have instilled programmes to replete iodine back into the food system, increasing cases of autoimmune thyroiditis are reported.[1]

Post-mortem studies, or studies performed after death, revealed that 27 percent of adult women, who during life did not know they had a problem, had evidence of chronic autoimmune thyroiditis. These studies also revealed a rise in the frequency of Hashimoto's thyroiditis over the past fifty years.[2] This could be proof that a person could go through life with an autoimmune thyroid condition and not even know it.

Subclinical hypothyroidism, defined as having an elevated TSH level and a normal T4 level, is usually the result of chronic autoimmune thyroiditis.[3] Various studies performed in England and the USA showed that 8 to 9 percent of people had subclinical hypothyroidism, respectively.[4,5]

A lot of these studies base their results on blood tests without any consideration for the symptoms one may experience. In my opinion, this is probably because it is difficult to gauge who has hypothyroidism based on symptoms simply because there are so many. Symptoms associated with hypothyroidism can easily be confused with symptoms of other disease states.

Based on the studies I have looked at and the clients I have seen throughout the years, I have a sneaking suspicion that the prevalence of hypothyroidism is highly under-reported.

Not-So-Common Symptoms of Hypothyroidism

One of the most frustrating things on my journey to discovering what was wrong with me was not having answers to the symptoms I was experiencing. I knew that the weight gain and fatigue stemmed from an underactive thyroid, however, some other symptoms were a complete mystery to me. Here, I have included *not-so-common* hypothyroid symptoms to be aware of so that you are better able to present a detailed medical history to your doctor. If I had known this information, it would have saved me a lot of heart-ache.

Symptoms you may not associate with hypothyroidism:

- Depression/Anxiety
- Inability to cope with low levels of stress
- Trouble falling or staying asleep
- Eczema/Acne/Psoriasis
- Hair loss or early loss of pigmentation of hair
- Difficulty with easy exercise programs
- High total cholesterol levels
- Increased sensitivity to many kinds of foods
- Gastrointestinal distress including bloating, cramping, gas, constipation and diarrhea

- Diseases of the gut like irritable bowel syndrome (IBS), gastritis, or Celiac's disease
- Pernicious (vitamin B12-deficient) or iron-deficient anemia
- Allergies

Feeling tired all the time, having difficulty losing weight, and feeling cold are the more common symptoms of hypothyroidism. The great thing is that a lot of these symptoms can be resolved with the right combination of medical and nutritional therapy. (Of course, I will only focus on the nutrition part).

Causes of Hypothyroidism

The truth is that there is a lot involved when it comes to understanding how the metabolic processes of hypothyroidism work. The production and use of thyroid hormones can go wrong under many different circumstances, thus making thyroid disease a lot more complicated than most people think.

Here are some examples of where thyroid metabolism could go wrong:

- The thyroid itself does not produce enough T4 and T3 (just to clarify, the thyroid produces more T4 than T3).

- T4 is predominantly converted to T3 in the liver. If the liver is not functioning properly, this process is inhibited. So you can imagine that if you have any kind of issue with your liver, thyroid metabolism will be compromised.

- T4 is also converted to T3 by a special enzyme produced in the intestines. If you have issues like bloating, indigestion, gas, cramping, diarrhea, or constipation, there is a good chance that this conversion is also compromised making less T3 available to metabolize.

- Selenium, an important trace mineral, is vital in converting T4 to T3. If you are deficient in selenium, this conversion will struggle to take place.

- Thyroid-binding globulin (TGB) is a protein responsible for binding with and transporting free active T3 hormone through the blood. If estrogen levels are too high, TBG proteins do not release T3 hormones to make them available for the body to use.

- You can become thyroid hormone resistant if too much free thyroid hormone is circulating in the blood. This means that the cells themselves will not receive the T3 that they need for metabolic functions.

- Your immune system can attack the thyroid tissue as a foreign object, rendering the thyroid unable to produce the proper amounts of thyroid hormones.[6]

To make matters more complicated, the immune system, the adrenal glands, and hormonal and blood-glucose regulation all play a role in thyroid function. Therefore, one must work with a qualified functional medicine practitioner or a doctor with a nutrition background to get a holistic picture of what is going on in the body before simply treating the thyroid itself.

Hashimoto's Thyroiditis

Believe it or not, 90 percent of thyroid issues are related to autoimmune disease. Hashimoto's disease is an autoimmune disease in which the immune system attacks healthy thyroid tissue. Although experts are not exactly sure what causes this autoimmune disease, there are many factors that are known to exacerbate the problem.

What are some of these factors?

- **An unhealthy gut.** Issues like irritable bowel syndrome (IBS), hypochloridia (decreased stomach acid), decreased motility of the gut (for example, constipation), or a "leaky" gut (increased intestinal permeability) can all contribute to an autoimmune attack.
- **Gluten.** Research has found that gluten contributes to a leaky gut and especially to autoimmune disorders of the thyroid and intestine.

- **Stress.** Stress puts extra strain on the adrenal glands to produce stress hormones like cortisol, epinephrine, and norepinephrine, which can cause a lot of damage if excessive amounts of them remain in the body over long periods of time. High-stress lifestyles can cause adrenal fatigue, which can also contribute to autoimmune disease.

- **Heavy metal poisoning**. Some people are more sensitive than others to heavy metals such as lead and mercury. These can also trigger an autoimmune response.

- **Highly processed diet**. A diet predominantly made up of refined grains and sugars offers little to no nutrition. Over time, this can also lead to autoimmune disease.

- **Bacterial infection**. Research shows that there is a connection between the bacteria *Yersinia enterocolitica* and Hashimoto's disease.

- **Candida.** This is a fungus that resides naturally within our intestines. However, an overgrowth can have deleterious effects on other organs, including the thyroid.

- **Parasites.** Studies from Europe, Australia, and the Middle East have found a connection between the common human intestinal parasite, *Blastocystis hominis* and IBS and hives (both of which are common issues in the early stages of Hashimoto's).[7]

How does the immune system end up attacking the thryroid?

Thyroid hormones are formed by thyroid peroxidase (TPO), an enzyme responsible for transforming iodide (the inactive form) to iodine (the active form). Excess hydrogen peroxide that is formed when creating iodine is cleared by the antioxidants selenium and glutathione peroxidase. The iodine is then attached to a thyroglobulin protein via the amino acid tyrosine in order to create T3 (triiodothyronine, 3 iodines attached to one thyroglobulin) and T4 (thyroxine, 4 iodines attached to one thyroglobulin).

Thyroid Hormone Production Made Easy:

Iodide +TPO = Iodine and,Hydrogen Peroxide

THEN

Hydrogen Peroxide + Selenium or Glutathione Peroxidase = Decreased Inflammation and,Healthy Thyroid Tissue

THEN

Iodine + Thyroglobulin protein + Tyrosine (an amino acid) = T3 or T4 hormones

In the presence of a selenium or glutathione peroxidase deficiency, the build-up of hydrogen peroxide can cause damage to the thyroid tissue. This triggers lymphocytes to enter the area of the thyroid tissue to repair the damage and causes inflammation. Unfortunately, this causes *further* damage. Thus, a vicious cycle is created that ultimately ends up in the demise of healthy thyroid tissue.

What are TPO and Thyroglobulin Antibodies?

Since TPO is the enzyme that ultimately causes oxidative stress and damage, the immune system creates antibodies against it in order to attack it. Ninety percent of people with Hashimoto's have elevated levels of TPO antibodies (TPOAb).

Thyroglobulin antibodies can also be formed. The body is more inclined to create antibodies against the thyroglobulin protein in the presence of excess iodine. Therefore, excess iodine can exacerbate or even trigger an autoimmune attack on the thyroid. (More on this in Chapter 5). Eighty percent of people with Hashimoto's have elevated thyroglobulin antibodies.

TPOAb above 30kU/L is indicative of Hashimoto's, TPOAb above 500kU/L is indicative of an aggressive autoimmune attack, and a TPOAb under 100kU/L is indicative of an autoimmune disorder but does not necessarily result in the development of hypothyroidism.[8]

CHAPTER 2

THE GUT CONNECTION

Thousands of years ago, a wise doctor named Hippocrates said that, "All disease begins in the gut." Fast-forward to modern day and exactly the same observation holds true. The digestive tract is the key to how food is digested, absorbed, and distributed to the cells for metabolic functions. If the digestive tract is not functioning properly, this ultimately leads to the breakdown of the body as a whole because vital nutrients do not get to the cells.

In my experience with clients, most people have issues with their digestive tracts. Whether the problem is reflux, stomach upset, or irritable bowel syndrome, the digestive process is somehow disrupted.

Signs that you may have issues with your digestive tract include the following:

- Bloating or gas
- Constipation or diarrhea

- Full feeling after eating only a little bit
- Reflux or gastro-esophogeal reflux disease (GERD)
- Food intolerances, especially to gluten and dairy
- Cramping or pain in your intestines

How the Digestive Process Works

Before getting into what a leaky gut is, it is important to understand how the digestive process works in order to grasp how important a well-functioning intestine is to optimal thyroid health. The following is a very simplistic breakdown, but it serves our purpose for explaining where things can go wrong. Let's take a look:

The mouth – The mouth is responsible for secreting saliva which holds the enzyme amylase. This particular enzyme starts the digestion process by breaking down carbohydrates. Vitamins and minerals B12, B6, C, and zinc can be absorbed here.

The stomach – The stomach secretes hydrochloric acid (HCl), which breaks down food so that digestive enzymes can break it down further. This is where proteins are broken down. Copper, iodine, fluoride and molybdenum can be absorbed here.

The small intestine – The small intestine is responsible for absorbing most of the nutrients our cells require for metabolism. More enzymes that digest proteins and fats are released here.

Pancreas- The pancreas is responsible for producing a lot of the digestive enzymes that are responsible for breaking down food (thus making it ready for absorption through the small intestine).

Liver – The liver produces bile, which is a liquid that contains enzymes needed to break down fats. It is also a liquid through which toxins and unnecessary substances are excreted out of the body.

Gall bladder – The gall bladder stores the bile produced by the liver until it is needed for fat breakdown.

The large intestine – The large intestine takes the food that could not be digested and removes it from the body. It is also host to a vast amount of bacteria that digest fibers that we cannot digest to produce nutrients that we need for optimal metabolic function. Vitamin K, biotin, sodium, potassium and chloride are absorbed here.

Now let's look at the digestive process again to see what happens when it deteriorates:

Mouth – The mouth may not produce enough saliva or amylase to start breaking down carbohydrates.

Stomach – For various reasons, the stomach may not secrete enough HCl or stomach acid. Decreased stomach acid can contribute to poor absorption of zinc, calcium, and iron. It can also cause failure to digest food properly, failure to sterilize stomach contents, increased allergies, and malabsorption of B12. Studies have shown a link between low stomach acid content and autoimmune thyroid disease.[4]

The small intestine – If food from the stomach is not sufficiently broken down, proper absorption of vitamins and minerals does not take place here. Undigested food serves as an ideal feeding ground for dangerous bacteria and parasites that further contribute to poor absorption of nutrients. An increased level of "bad" bacteria in the intestine is referred to as small intestinal bacterial overgrowth (SIBO) and can result from decreased stomach acid, decreased small intestinal motility (in other words, the small intestine does not move fast enough), or decreased immunity.

Pancreas – The pancreas may not secrete enough enzymes for the sufficient breakdown of food in the small intestine. Diseases like celiac disease and Crohn's disease can cause pancreatic insufficiency.[6] Again, this adds to the feeding ground for bad bacteria and parasites.

Liver – In the case of a leaky gut, the liver works harder to excrete toxins from the body. As a result, more toxic bile filled with free radicals is produced, which can further increase intestinal permeability. (I will explain what this means in a bit). This bile can be refluxed into the pancreas and can be the cause of pancreatic disease. There is evidence that there is a greater chance for liver toxicity due to increased permeability of the gut (or leaky gut).

Gall bladder – A sluggish gall bladder interferes with the liver's ability to get rid of toxins. Hypothyroidism can actually cause a sluggish gall bladder.

The large intestine – Nutrients absorbed here may not be properly absorbed. Vitamin K which is an essential nutrient for bone health and immunity, may decrease in the blood. Undigested foods may remain here, further exacerbating issues like IBS and abdominal discomfort.

What Affects Our Gastro-intestinal Tract Negatively?

- **Use of proton pump inhibitors like Nexium or Prilosec.** According to Dr. Izabella Wentz, a doctor of pharmacy and an author of the book, *Hashimoto's Thyroiditis, Lifestyle Interventions for Finding and Treating the Root Cause*, these drugs are over-prescribed for issues such as GERD. They decrease the amount of stomach acid found in the stomach resulting in disaster for proper breakdown and absorption of nutrients and the possibility of build-up of dangerous bacteria in the intestinal tract.

- **Diet full of sugar and processed grains.** Sugar is an easy way to feed unwanted bacteria and gluten from processed grains exacerbates a leaky gut.

- **Antibiotics.** Sure, antibiotics have helped us to recover and have protected us from possible dangerous illnesses. However, with too much exposure to antibiotics, the delicate balance of good and bad bacteria is disrupted.

- **Oral contraceptives.** There is research showing that the birth control pill can cause changes in beneficial bacterial and cause nutrient depletions. In fact, oral contraception is one of the reasons autoimmune disease is more common in women than men.

What is the lesson to be learned here? Most chronic disease has its roots in a dysfunctional digestive tract **and thyroid disease is no exception.**

What Is a Leaky Gut?

When people hear the term "leaky gut," they might be disgusted envisioning disturbing images in the bathroom. What leaky gut refers to, however, is increased intestinal permeability. One of the functions of the intestine is to provide a barrier between toxins, bacteria and proteins that can exist without causing

24

harm in the gut, but not in the body and the rest of the body. With factors such as the use of medications like proton-pump inhibitors, eating a highly processed diet and the overuse of antibiotics, this barrier can break down, the integrity of the intestinal lining can be compromised and substances that are not supposed to enter the body can make their way through.

For the purpose of explaining a leaky gut in a simple manner, let's imagine that the intestinal lining is made up of structures that are called villi and tight junctions. You can think of the villi as the "fingers" of the intestinal wall that absorb nutrients. The tight junctions are like a cloth strainer that fits above these so-called fingers. When you strain foods in the kitchen, food that is small enough goes through whereas bigger bits of food remain in the strainer. This is what the tight junctions of the intestines do for the villi. They stop bigger, dangerous substances from being absorbed into the bloodstream. This function of the small intestine, keeping bigger particles (like bacteria) inside and absorbing small particles (like nutrients) is one of the most important for maintaining health.

If something compromises the integrity of the gut wall, the strainer (aka tight junctions) is broken and bigger particles pass through to the bloodstream. The body does not recognize these bigger particles and calls on the immune system to get rid of them. The problem with this is that if this happens often enough, the immune system goes awry and can send its "soldiers" to attack perfectly healthy tissues like the thyroid. (Therefore, ultimately, Hashimoto's thyroiditis is not really a problem of the thyroid gland but of a dysfunctional immune system.)

Why do tight junctions break down? There are many reasons. To give an example, one of the biggest contributing dietary factors to breaking down the tight junctions of the intestine is gluten.

Dr. Alessio Fasano, a pioneer in Celiac disease and intestinal permeability research, discovered the regulating molecules responsible for opening and closing tight junctions. According to Dr. Fasano, zonulin is released in everyone when there is small intestinal bacterial overgrowth (SIBO) and when there is gluten available in the diet. The gliadin part of gluten causes zonulin release in the gut.

Let me emphasize this point: gluten opens the tight junctions in *everyone*, not just in people with thyroid or autoimmune disease. This fact is important to remember when we talk about the benefits of applying a gluten-free lifestyle in subsequent chapters.

Diseases or conditions associated with leaky gut
- Inflammatory and infectious bowel diseases - Chronic inflammatory arthritides - Acne, psoriasis - Eczema - IBS - AIDS - Chronic hepatitis - Chronic pancreatitis - Cystic fibrosis[8]

Leaky Gut and Autoimmune Disease

As you can see, autoimmune disease can be a huge possibility in sensitive people (by "sensitive people," I mean those who have the genetic predisposition to develop an autoimmune disorder).

A 2012 review of research on leaky gut and autoimmune disease stated that there is a correlation between how the intestine is functioning and whether or not an autoimmune response will take place.[11] Also, although genetic predisposition can play a role, the research suggests that an autoimmune response can be reversed if the environmental trigger is taken away.

What does this mean? It means that if you take away what is causing an immune attack to take place, you could send an autoimmune disease into remission. Celiac disease is a great example of this. When gluten is removed from the diet of people suffering from Celiac disease, an autoimmune disease that attacks the small intestine, symptoms and biomarkers associated with the disease are vastly improved.

There is evidence of this with other autoimmune diseases as well, especially Hashimoto's thyroiditis. When gluten is removed from their diet, many people with hypothyroidism see a marked improvement in their health.

There is still a lot of research that needs to be done before I can provide more conclusive recommendations. However, the finding that removing an environmental trigger could improve symptoms of or even heal an autoimmune disorder is significant in creating a therapy protocol for diseases such as Hashimoto's thyroiditis.

The Importance of the Microbiome

According to Dr. Robynne Chutkan, an integrative gastroenterologist and founder and CEO of Gutbliss, we are host to an entire ecosystem referred to as the microbiome. Bacteria, viruses and parasites are all part of this complex microbiota and there is a symbiosis between us and them. However, this microbiome has been altered to the point where increased disease is seen. This is so because of the very "clean" lifestyle we are used to today, with the use of antiseptic cleansers and hand washes, the increasing use of antibiotics and a lack of exposure to nature.

There has been an explosion of research in recent years that emphasises the importance of the diversity of the microbiome. Different bacterial strains help to produce metabolites which can positively or negatively impact the intestines, the brain, the liver and the immune system. The one factor that directly influences the health of the microbiome is diet. Eating a highly processed diet leads to a decrease in the biodiversity of the microbiome and has been documented to contribute to disease states such as inflammatory bowel disease (IBD), irritable bowel syndrome (IBS), cancer, diabetes and asthma.[12] Gram-negative or "bad" bacteria have also been shown to contribute to the pathogenesis of hypothyroidism by inhibiting the conversion of T4 to T3 in the liver.[13]

Conversely, a diet rich in specific fibers from fruits and vegetables can improve the microbiome and therefore have a positive effect on health. An example of this can be seen with the production of short chain fatty acids by bacteria that inhabit the colon or large intestine. The bacteria feed off of dietary fiber and produce short chain fatty acids which in turn reduce pathogenic bacteria and potentially regulate genes that are involved with immune and metabolic diseases. Research shows that short chain fatty acids and T3 (the active form of thyroid hormone) cooperate in maintaining proper intestinal health. Lactobacillus and Bifidobacteria are both probiotic strains that can enhance short fatty acid production.[14, 15, 16, 17, 18,19]

Specific bacteria have also been shown to improve thyroid function in animal studies. *L. reuteri* supplementation increased free T4 levels in mice. These mice were also slimmer, more active and had healthier skin than control mice, which correlated with free T4 levels.[20] This research is promising because it further supports the theory that the microbiome composition may affect endocrine and immunological systems. In other words, the microbiome may have a big impact on the health of your thyroid and is directly affected by the foods you eat.

SIBO – Small Intestine Bacterial Overgrowth

Just as a good microbiome can support health, a bad one can be deleterious to us. Very simply, when there is an imbalance between "good" and "bad" bacteria, this contributes to the development of a leaky gut.

Small intestinal bacterial overgrowth (SIBO for short) can

complicate therapies that are used to heal the digestive tract. It is defined as an overgrowth of gram-negative, anaerobic bacterial strains in the small intestine (which are not present in a healthy intestine). It is more likely in people that have motility issues caused by things such as IBS, diabetes or certain medications.[21] As stated by Dr. Fasano, bacterial overgrowth increases intestinal permeability. Therefore, if you do have SIBO, it is imperative that proper action is taken to get rid of it.

As you can see, it is very important to emphasize the microbiome and to learn about the pivotal role that nutrition can play in changing it to enhance health.

Nutrition Considerations for Candida *albicans* and *Helicobacter pylori*

From my experience, two common issues that I came across among my patients and that needed to be addressed in order to heal the gut were a fungal overgrowth of Candida albicans or a bacterial infection of Helicobacter pylori. Understanding what these are and finding ways to treat them nutritionally, is very important for the optimal functioning of the digestive tract.

Candida albicans

Candida albicans is a fungus that can have a symbiotic relationship with healthy individuals. What this means is that we help it out by providing it with a home and food and it helps us by contributing to nutrient absorption and digestion. However, when there is an overgrowth of *Candida albicans*, it has the ability to escape by breaking down the intestinal walls and thus contributing to a leaky gut. When this happens, it can turn pathogenic and cause serious fungal infections.

In patients with autoimmune diseases like Hashimoto's thyroiditis, the number of *Candida albicans* antibodies in the cells can be six times higher than in those of healthy individuals.[22] There is speculation that *Candida albicans* overgrowth can even contribute to the formation of autoimmune diseases. However, further research needs to be done in order to confirm this.

What causes a *Candida albicans* overgrowth?

1. Antibiotics: When you do a course of antibiotics, you not only kill the bacteria that cause infection, you also kill the good bacteria that protect the immune system. Therefore, if you do not replace the good bacteria, they cannot protect you against an overgrowth of *Candida albicans*.

2. Birth control pill: If you have a diminished microbiome and have a weakened immune system, the pill can also contribute to yeast infections.

3. Oral corticosteroids: People with asthma who take inhalants are at increased risk of developing candidiasis in the mouth, which can lead to systemic infection.[24]

4. Cancer patients: Candidiasis can be invasive in people with cancer and can cause serious complications.[25]

5. Diabetes: In people who have Type 1 or Type 2 diabetes, the increased amount of sugar available in their tissues means that they are at a higher risk for developing a yeast infection, because sugar is a primary food source for *Candida albicans.*

6. Weakened immune system: Obviously, if the immune system isn't working properly, you are at higher risk for developing a *Candida albicans* infection.[26] As mentioned previously, one example of an illness that can weaken the immune system and increase risk of infection is Hashimoto's thyroiditis.

Symptoms of a Candida infection include the following:

- Chronic fatigue
- Mood disorders
- Recurring vaginal and urinary tract infection
- Oral thrush

- Sinus infections
- Brain fog
- Skin and nail fungal infections
- Hormonal imbalance

A protocol for healing the gut should definitely include a plan to get rid of a fungal infection if one is present.

If you have *Candida*.

The protocol to get rid of a *Candida* infection can be quite strict. However, it is worth it when considering the benefits of better health. In general, *Candida albicans* feed on sugar. Therefore, a diet low in simple sugars and carbohydrates is warranted here. Foods like grains, potatoes, beans, lentils, legumes and some fruits should be avoided when following a *Candida* elimination protocol.

The foods that must be avoided when tackling a *Candida* overgrowth are also the ones to avoid when following an autoimmune protocol to reduce symptoms associated with an autoimmune condition such as Hashimoto's thyroiditis. This will be discussed in more detail in chapter 5.

Helicobacter pylori

Helicobacter pylori is one of the most prevalent global pathogens and can lead to gastrointestinal diseases such as peptic ulcers and several stomach cancers. In fact, 50 percent of the world has *H. pylori* present in their bodies.[29] Unfortunately, this pathogen is increasingly resistant to antibiotics, and more research needs to be done in order to establish better antibiotic and alternative treatment protocols for patients who may be resistant.

There is research that supports a positive association between *H.pylori* and thyroid nodules in a euthyroid in people with no thyroid problems (the euthyroid population).[30] This could suggest a role for *H.pylori* in the disease progression of hypothyroidism.

At a minimum, an overgrowth of *H.pylori* can cause chronic gastritis. When it comes to healing the gut, this should definitely be addressed with your physician.

If you have H.pylori, consider the following foods:

Cranberries.

Cranberries are small red berries that have been proven to have a therapeutic effect against urinary tract infections. This is because they contain a substance called proanthocyanidins which decrease the binding of infectious bacteria to the tissue lining.

Some research has shown that cranberries may also contribute to the eradication of *H.pylori*. A study done on animals found that 80percent of mice infected with *H.pylori* and given cranberry juice were cured. An eradication rate of 20 percent was seen four week post-therapy.[31]

A few human studies have also explored the potential of cranberry juice to fight *H.pylori*. One study showed that the inclusion of cranberry juice in a standardized antibiotic protocol to fight *H.pylori* may improve eradication rates in females.[32] Another study showed that cranberry juice was able to manage *H.pylori* colonization in asymptomatic children.[33]

Further research is needed to understand how cranberries actually decrease *H.pylori* and how to use cranberries in treatment protocols. However, cranberries do show promise as an option to help with eradication.

Berries in general are great in the fight against *H.pylori*. Blueberries, bilberries, elderberries, raspberries and strawberries all inhibit *H.pylori* and enhance the susceptibility of *H.pylori* to clarithromycin (a common antibiotic used against *H.pylori*). What this means is that if you eat berries while on antibiotics, the treatment will be more effective than if you take the antibiotics on their own.

Curcumin.

Curcumin is extracted from turmeric and has anti-inflammatory, antioxidant and anti-infectious properties. It also helps the liver with the process of detoxifying the body.

In terms of *H.pylori*, an animal study done in 2011 showed that curcumin was able to eradicate the bacteria in mice.[34] More research needs to be done to ascertain if curcumin is as effective on humans.

Indirectly, curcumin may eradicate or alleviate *H.pylori* by having a therapeutic effect on stomach ulcers (many of which are caused by *H.pylori* infection). A study was done to assess the effectiveness of curcumin on stomach ulcers.

Three hundred milligrams of turmeric were given five times a day to ulcer patients. After four weeks, 48 percent of these patients had no ulcers, and after another 12 twelve weeks, 76 percent had no ulcers.[35] This may justify curcumin as an alternative therapy for stomach ulcers.

Ginger.

Traditionally, ginger has been used to alleviate many issues that have to do with gastric distress. Things like nausea, ulcers, motion sickness, inflammatory disorders and hyperemesis gravidarum (a fancy word for excessive vomiting) are all issues for which ginger has been used.

A study showed that ginger extracts and gingerols were able to inhibit the development of *H.pylori* in vitro (in a lab).[36] However, this study may also suggest that gingerols may be effective in preventing or treating *H.pylori* in vivo (in live subjects).

Another study researching *H.pylori* in Mongolian gerbils noted that ginger prevented and treated the bacteria.[37]

Ginger is another food that can be considered an alternative therapy for treating gastro-intestinal distress.

Mastic gum.

I am particularly proud of this food as it comes from a plant that is native to the Greek island of Chios. Since 3000 BC, mastic gum has been used by the Greeks in cooking, in cosmetics and in treating gastric illnesses.

Mastic is a gum-like substance that comes from the stem of the tree *Pistacia lentiscus*. There are animal and now some human studies that have shown mastic gum to improve gastric secretions and reduce and treat gastro-intestinal ulcers. In a double-blind controlled clinical study, one gram of mastic gum per day was able to reduce the size of ulcers in most patients.[38,39]

Research from the *New England Journal of Medicine* showed that mastic gum, even in very low doses, is very effective at killing *H. pylori*.[40]

A 2011 study found that mastic gum was able to abolish *H.pylori* in vitro.[41] Some in vivo studies confirmed this as well. In a study published in 2010, two groups were given mastic gum to treat *H. pylori*. One group of thirteen patients received 350 mg of mastic gum three times a day. The other group of thirteen patients was given 1.05 grams of mastic gum for fourteen days. *H.pylori* eradication was seen in four of thirteen and five of thirteen patients, respectively.[42]

As always, more research needs to be done to confirm which constituents of mastic gum have anti-bacterial activity, and the mechanisms through which they work.

Broccoli sprouts.

Isothiocyanate sulforaphane, an important constituent of broccoli sprouts, is being studied for its various protective effects against chronic diseases. It also has a very potent and selective antibacterial activity against *H.pylori*. Because this substance is also an anti-inflammatory, it works systemically (or throughout the body) to reduce the symptoms of *H.pylori* infection.

In Japan, broccoli sprouts with high concentrations of the sulforaphane precursor, glucoraphanin, were given to *H.Pylori* positive adults for two months. There were significant reductions in markers of inflammation and *H.pylori* levels. Interestingly, these results disappeared at the end of the intervention.[45] In 2014, a similar study took place in Iran and had similar results.[46]

Cabbage juice, moringa (leaves of a certain tree), okra and some types of seaweed also show activity against H.pylori.

Probiotics

A meta-analysis which looked at thirty-three clinical studies of the effect of probiotic supplements on *H.pylori* concluded that there was a higher eradicating effect in the groups that took probiotics than in the groups that did not.

Various strains have also been tested for their effect on *H.pylori*. Lactobacillus and *Saccharomyces boulardii* have both been shown to be active against the bacteria.[47,48]

In 2005, a consensus conference was held to talk about the diet-related therapies that could be used to protect against or to ameliorate *H.pylori* infections. The participants concluded that efforts to use a diet-based approach to reduce *H.pylori* infection may be more attractive in terms of cost, treatment, tolerability and cultural acceptability.

Also, given that there is an increasing bacterial resistance to antibiotics, using diet to decrease *H.pylori* infection and associated symptoms instead of completely eradicating it may be more beneficial for human health. This is so because as a lot of research shows today, the diversity of the microbiome is essential to enhancing the immune system and protecting against disease.

In my humble opinion, if a doctor prescribes antibiotics to get rid of *H.pylori*, dietary-driven lifestyle changes should also be made in order to protect against further infection. All of the foods I have mentioned that help to reduce *H.pylori* infection are also foods that should be included in a healthy meal plan for treating hypothyroidism anyway. Berries provide powerful antioxidants that support the immune system, ginger and mastic gum help the digestive process, curcumin helps with detoxification and immune system modulation, broccoli also aids the detoxification process and supports the function of the liver and probiotics help to maintain a balanced bacterial diversity that ultimately protects us from illness.

Obviously, more research needs to be done in order to come up with specific nutrition protocols to fight *H.pylori* infections.

However, the research that *has* been done shows a lot of promise.

What Does a Leaky Gut Have to Do with Proper Thyroid Function?

As discussed previously, there is a connection between a leaky gut and autoimmune disease and apparently, gluten can play a role in this activity. How exactly is the thyroid affected when someone suffers from a compromised gut?

Well, in the case of Hashimoto's disease, a leaky gut makes sense because Hashimoto's is, in and of itself an autoimmune disorder. However, is there evidence to conclude that a leaky gut can affect people with hypothyroidism without any indication of an autoimmune problem?

As usual, the answer is not clear cut. This is because not only can a low-functioning intestine influence the thyroid but a low-functioning thyroid can also influence the gut. Here are a few examples:

- The gut is responsible for assisting T4 (the inactive form of thyroid hormone) to turn into T3 (the active form of thyroid hormone). This is done with the help of an enzyme called intestinal sulfatase. This enzyme is produced by the good bacteria found in the gut. (Remember, a good microbiome enhances health!) Therefore, if there is an imbalance between healthy bacteria and unhealthy bacteria, this enzyme could be compromised and therefore also the production of the active form of thyroid hormone.

- Inflammation in the gut increases cortisol (or stress hormones) which reduces the active thyroid hormone T3.

- The cell walls of gut bacteria, called lipopolysaccharides, negatively affect thyroid metabolism by reducing thyroid hormone levels, dulling thyroid hormone receptor sites, increasing amounts of inactive T3, decreasing thyroid-stimulating hormone (TSH) and promoting autoimmune thyroid disease.

- Constipation also contributes to a decrease in thyroid metabolism, as it increases the amount of estrogen that remains in the intestine. This decreases the amount of free active thyroid hormone available to be used by the cells. Also, conversely, not having enough thyroid hormone causes constipation.

So, as one can see, the thyroid and the gut are interconnected and work together to optimize metabolism. If either is compromised, problems will occur. This is why it is just as important to address healing the intestine as it is to support the thyroid nutritionally in order for the body to work optimally.

Pathways to Healing the Gut

There are a few simple things everyone can do to increase their gut health. In my experience, *everyone* can benefit from following a protocol to heal the digestive tract. Remember that each person is different and the following are only general guidelines. If you would like a protocol specific to you, contact a functional medicine practitioner in your area who can help you on your path to healing.

Eliminate Inflammatory Foods

The first step to healing the gut is to get rid of foods that exacerbate the condition. These foods are different for everyone, but included below are the main culprits that research has shown to affect most people negatively:

Avoid grains. Gliadin, a component of the protein part of gluten, is responsible for stimulating zonulin secretion (which increases intestinal permeability).[49] It is very important to stay away from grains containing gluten in order to heal the gut, especially for people with Hashimoto's thyroiditis or another autoimmune condition. These foods include wheat, barley, rye, spelt and oats. Depending on the severity of one's symptoms, all flours and foods like rice and corn should be avoided. If you really want to heal, abstain from these foods altogether until you begin to see improvement. Afterward, you can reintroduce sprouted versions of organic grains one to two times per week.

Avoid soy products. Soy is well known for being a genetically-modified crop. Unfortunately, unfermented soy is linked to *many* disease states that have impaired gut function.[50] These include thyroid issues, digestive distress and hormonal imbalance. When included in food in a very processed state (an example is a common food additive called soy lecithin), soy can increase estrogen levels (which, as I said before, can decrease the function of thyroid hormones) and can cause gastrointestinal issues, as it is not well tolerated by the gut. Make sure to avoid soy products, including soy milk, and check food labels for additives like soy lecithin.

Avoid conventional dairy or all dairy. If you do not know where your milk is coming from, it is safe to say that you do not know what techniques are being used to produce that milk. For example, antibiotics may have been given to conventional dairy cows to decrease disease, or the cows may have been fed with genetically-modified grains. Buying raw milk from a local producer can make you certain that you are getting milk from grass-fed cows. Having a relationship with local producers also holds them accountable for how they are taking care of their livestock.

Again, depending on the severity of the problem, you may need to avoid dairy products altogether.

Avoid processed foods. It goes without saying that steering clear from any processed food is of absolute importance at this time. Processed foods are full of the additives and chemicals that probably added to the cause of your thyroid problem. So, a good rule of thumb is that if it comes in a box and has more than three ingredients, ***don't eat it***. Stick to real, whole foods that will give you the nutrition you need to get healthy.

Introduce Real Foods

Organic vegetables. When trying to heal the gut, choose organic fruits and vegetables that are void of any pesticides and insecticides. It is well documented that these chemicals cause endocrine dysfunction and hormonal imbalance.

The US Environmental Working Group publishes a list of the fruits and vegetables that are known to have the most exposure to insecticides and pesticides. You can find these foods under "The Dirty Dozen". When choosing produce from this list, you should always opt for organic. You can also take a look at the Clean Fifteen list. From this group of fruits and vegetables, you don't necessarily have to buy organic. Simply put one to two shots of vinegar in a bowl of water and allow the fruits and vegetables you will use to sit in this water for fifteen minutes.

Decreasing the intestines' exposure to chemicals helps to decrease inflammation.

Vegetables should be steamed in order to break down phytic acid and to decrease further damage to an inflamed gut. Steaming also decreases the goitrogens which inhibit iodine uptake by the thyroid. (Goitrogens are found in cruciferous vegetables such as sweet potato, broccoli and cauliflower.) Try to avoid raw vegetables at this time if they cause a problem for you.

Organic fruits. The main form of sugar in your diet should come from fruit. Although fructose has gotten a bad reputation in the past, recent research suggests that fructose can help to decrease the production of cortisol (a stress hormone). Research has also shown that fructose can be "cytoprotective" and can protect liver cells in a low oxygen environment.[51,52,53,54]

Again, if raw fruit is not well tolerated, it may be wise to eat apple and pear purees until there is improvement in gut function.

Healthy fats: Saturated fat is making a comeback. Research now shows us that saturated fats help to reduce the adaptive response of the body to stress.[55] In the case of intestinal permeability, saturated fats help to protect the lining of the intestine and therefore decrease the chances of a leaky gut as compared to unsaturated fats.[56] (To find out more, check out chapter 5).

The Magic of Bone Broth

There has been a lot of hype about bone broth as a magical remedy. There are Paleo followers that swear by it, but at the same time, there are many vegans and vegetarians who completely disagree with using bone broth as a means to healing. As a nutritionist, I am not here to try and sell you a lifestyle (Paleo or Vegan). I am here to offer the science behind why certain foods may be beneficial for specific ailments. At the end of the day, how you use this information is up to you. So, let's explore the science behind bone broth.

Bone broth is not something new. It has been used for many years by many different cultures. Bones, ribs, feet and anything with more cartilage have been used to create stocks as a base for soups and other recipes.

Here is what bone broth contains and why certain of its constituents can help with healing (in this case, the gut).

Cartilage

The joint cartilage is the kind that is incorporated into broth. Studies have found that ingesting cartilage drastically improves degenerative joint disease and inflammatory bowel disease.

Cartilage supplementation also increases the function of B, T and macrophage immune cells. Since 80 percent of the immune system can be found in the gastrointestinal lining, supporting the gut and the immune system with cartilage supplementation is definitely beneficial.

What cartilage can help with. Degenerative joint disease, inflammatory bowel disease, gut repair, immune support

Collagen and Gelatin

Collagen and gelatin are one in the same. Collagen comes from the Greek word, kola, which means to glue together. And this is exactly what it does in the body. One fourth of the protein found in the body is in the form of collagen. It is needed for healthy gums, younger looking skin and arterial health. Gelatin describes the collagen extracted from bone broth.

Gelatin

Gelatin has been studied since the early 1800s for the treatment of various medical conditions. Most research has shown gelatin's ability to aid in digestion, specifically with the digestion of milk products, beans and meat. Experts therefore recommended that it be added to baby formula. An interesting find in this early research was that gelatin is able to increase the body's ultilization of gluten.

Gelatin also helps with hyper- or hypochloridia (increased or decreased stomach acid).

Chinese studies have shown gelatin to increase red blood cell and hemoglobin count, increase serum calcium level, increase the absorption and utilization of calcium and prevent and treat myotonia atrophica (muscle wasting).

What gelatin can help with. Digestion, low stomach acid, increased absorption of minerals, muscle wasting

Collagen.

Collagen is made up of three specific amino acids: glycine, proline and lysine. Vitamin C is also vital to the synthesis of collagen. Let's take a deeper look at what the research says on these important amino acids.

Glycine

The amino acid glycine has many functions in the body. Some functions are listed below:

- It helps to make other amino acids.
- It is a primary ingredient of heme, the part of the blood that carries oxygen throughout the body.
- It is used in the synthesis of creatine which is important for energy production.

- It contributes to the synthesis of bile salts.
- It helps to form DNA
- It is used in phase 1 detoxification in the liver and helps to form glutathione which is an antioxidant used for phase 2 detoxification.
- It affects the stabilization of blood glucose as it helps to form glucose from protein sources in times of fasting.

Research shows that glycine can also help with the following conditions:

- It's associated with a reduced risk of asthma.
- It stimulates gastric acid secretion.
- It increases wound healing.
- It helps with liver problems such as jaundice.
- It helps with detoxification processes.
- If taken during a fast, it prevents degeneration.

Proline

One of proline's main roles is in the structure of collagen. Therefore, it is an important part of connective tissue and it decreases in the body if it is not taken in through the diet (even though the body can manufacture proline by itself). Proline is also beneficial in increasing memory and preventing depression.

Lysine

Lysine is commonly known as the antiviral protein. It is used to fight off viral infections like herpes simplex. It is an essential amino acid, which means that it is not produced by the body and it must be acquired from the diet.

Lysine has many functions, one of which is that it is used to produce carnitine which is used by the body to burn fat and decrease cholesterol. It also increases the absorption of calcium and is needed to produce collagen. Lysine is therefore very important for bone, skin, hair, nail and cardiac health.

On average, a person needs 12 milligrams of lysine per kilogram of weight per day for good health. Therefore, a person who weighs 70 kilos would need 840 milligrams per day. One hundred grams of bone broth contains 4.4 grams of lysine. Therefore, you would get a good dose of lysine from only a small portion of bone broth.

It is important to remember that lysine fights for absorption through the intestine with arginine. Therefore, if there is too much arginine in the diet, lysine needs to be supplemented in order to have a therapeutic effect.

Minerals Found in Bone Broth:

Calcium, phosphorous and magnesium are all important minerals that are found in bone broth. They are all involved in supporting bone health as well as a healthy metabolism. It is common for people with hypothyroidism to have calcium and magnesium deficiencies, and therefore supplementing the diet with bone broth is a great way to add these important minerals to the diet.

As you can see, bone broth is beneficial for various ailments, but it is an especially important food for healing and restoring the gut. I typically recommend two cups of bone broth per day, one on an empty stomach in the morning and one in the evening a few hours before bedtime.

You can make bone broths from organic beef or chicken. It's typically better to use bones that have more cartilage like those from the ribs. In addition to drinking bone broth you can also use it in soups or other dishes.

Dairy – To Eat or Not to Eat?

There is a lot of controversy regarding whether dairy products are, in fact, essential to one's diet. Foods like milk, cheese, yogurt and butter are high in calcium, vitamin B12 and magnesium and can provide beneficial bacteria that are needed by the gut to support gastrointestinal functioning as well as the immune system.

However, many people do not tolerate dairy products as they are difficult to digest. In my experience with patients with hypothyroidism, many do, in fact, have an intolerance to casein, which is the main protein found in dairy. Anecdotally, hypothyroid patients who have cut dairy from their diet have seen improvements with issues such as reflux, irritable bowel syndrome, arthritic pain, asthma and excess phlegm.

When one has a leaky gut, casein can escape into the bloodstream and can trigger the immune system to destroy it as a foreign invader. Since this is the case, it can also be a trigger for an autoimmune attack against the thyroid.

Therefore, when administering a protocol to heal the gut, I exclude dairy initially and have people incorporate it into their diet only after some time, to see if it is tolerated.

When I do reintroduce dairy, I recommend that people use organic dairy products as well as goat's or sheep's milk, as it is typically better tolerated than cow's milk.[58] However, the casein protein from goat's or sheep's milk is very similar to that found in cow's milk, and a lot of hypothyroid patients still need to exclude these forms of dairy from their diet in order to see improved symptoms.

Raw versus Conventional Dairy

It is also important to make the distinction between raw dairy products and conventional dairy products. According to Chris Kresser, a well-known functional medicine practitioner, raw dairy seems to be superior in vitamin and mineral content than conventional dairy products. There is not yet enough conclusive data, but Kresser also claims that there is anecdotal evidence that seems to show that raw milk is better tolerated by individuals than is conventional milk.

However, if you have been eating conventional dairy products for a while (as many of us have because they are a staple in a Westernized diet), chances are that you will be sensitive to raw dairy products as well.

There is also some evidence that different types of casein from different types of animals cause inflammation. A1 casein typically causes inflammation whereas A2 casein does not.[60] Therefore, hypothetically, drinking milk from A2 cows may not cause a reaction. However, more research needs to be done to confirm this.

Again, in most cases, dairy should be excluded altogether when healing the gut. In my experience, many people do not tolerate dairy at all and need to exclude it from their diet entirely. It is important to work with a functional nutritionist or doctor to figure out what your body can tolerate and what it cannot.

Supplements that May Help with Healing the Gut:

The following are some natural food supplements that are commonly used in some detox regimes designed to heal the gut. Below, I present some research that helps to support their use.

Black walnut.

Black walnut is used to treat parasitic worm infections as well as diseases like syphilis, diphtheria and leukemia.[61,62,63]

In the context of healing the gut, killing any unwanted parasites is key to allowing the gut to work optimally. Think of it this way: if parasites are eating up all of the good nutrition you put into healing your gut, you won't really heal your gut in the end.

Therefore, I recommend that you include some black walnuts in any protocol for healing the intestines.

Pau d'arco.

Pau d'arco comes from the bark of a tree. It has many healing qualities, including the fact that it decreases arthritic pain, fights *Candida*, reduces inflammation, heals ulcers, fights cancer, has anti-viral and anti-fungal properties and acts as a natural laxative.[64,65,66]

Pau d'arco contains a natural and very potent antioxidant called beta-lapachone, which has wound healing activity and helps to fight cancers.[67,68]

With its potent antioxidant and other antibacterial and antiviral properties, Pau d'Arco is also a great natural food to add to a protocol for healing the gut.

Cascara sagrada.

Cascara sagrada is a tree bark that is well-documented for its natural laxative effects. The bark contains chemicals called anthraquinones which react with intestinal bacteria to stimulate the bowels. There has also been some research showing that it helps to fight cancer and some ailments such as gallstones.

There are additional supplements that your doctor or functional medicine practitioner may use to enhance a protocol for healing the gut. I discuss a few of these here:

Hydrochloric acid (HCl).

As mentioned before, stomach acid is vital for the proper breakdown of foods and for protecting against dangerous bacteria entering the intestine. If you have performed the proper tests and know that you do not produce enough stomach acid, an HCl betaine supplement can help you. Remember, if you do not have enough gastric acid, this could contribute to small intestinal bacterial overgrowth (SIBO), which compromises your ability to absorb nutrients, decreases your immunity, and exacerbates autoimmune disease.

According to Dr. Jonathan Wright, author of *Why Stomach Acid Is Good for You*, low levels of stomach acid are responsible for a myriad of issues including hair loss, blood sugar control, allergies, autoimmune disease, neurological disorders and thyroid dysfunction. Obviously, more substantial research needs to be undertaken. However, it makes sense that if you do not break down your food properly, the digestive process is compromised and nutrient deficiencies are inevitable as a result.

If an HCl betaine supplement is appropriate for you, make sure to look for one with added pepsin, the enzyme responsible for breaking down protein in the stomach. People with low stomach acid typically have low levels of pepsin as well. It is then advisable to start with a low dose, 1-2 pills (about 650 mg or less each), taken at the beginning of each meal. You increase the dose by 1 pill every 2 days until you feel a burning sensation in your stomach or belly button area shortly after taking the HCl. Your proper dose is the last dose taken before the burning sensation occurred. For example, if you feel the burning sensation at seven pills, taking six pills per meal is your proper dose.

It goes without saying that taking HCl supplements should not be ventured upon alone. Please seek advice from a trained functional medicine practitioner to help you determine if this treatment is appropriate for you and what the correct dosage is.

Natural Ways to Boost Stomach Acid:

Bone Broth

Although there is no research to show that bone broth increases stomach acid, it can help to boost the health of the stomach in order to allow it to withstand the amount of stomach acid needed to absorb nutrients and to maintain health. In addition to its many healing properties, research has shown that bone broth helps to prevent ulcers as it is rich in glycine and proline which are amino acids that protect the mucosal lining of the stomach.

Lemon and Apple Cider Vinegar

These foods are traditional remedies that have been used throughout the years to help with issues such as GERD and indigestion. Both lemon and apple cider vinegar have been found to have health benefits, such as decreasing oxidative stress in the body. However, there is limited research to determine their ability to increase stomach acid.

Digestive Bitters

Unfortunately, controlled studies need to be performed in order to confirm the therapeutic use of digestive bitters in digestive issues, however, some studies have shown that digestive bitters have the ability to increase the flow of digestive juices, including HCl.

Here is a list of some of them used in Chinese and Western medicine:

- Barberry bark
- Caraway
- Dandelion
- Fennel
- Gentian root
- Ginger
- Globe artichoke
- Goldenseal root
- Hops
- Milk thistle
- Peppermint
- Wormwood
- Yellow dock

Ideally, it would be good to visit a qualified herbalist that could prescribe the right mixture of herbs for your particular condition.

Digestive Enzymes

Did you know that by the time you turn forty, your enzyme production could be 25 percent less than what it was when you were a child? Digestive enzymes further help to break food down decreasing the chances of an extra feeding ground for bad bacteria and enhancing the amount of nutrients you absorb.

Enzymes not only help us to properly digest and therefore absorb our food, but they also work systemically to reduce inflammation (an added plus for healing the gut).

Here is a run-down of common enzymes:

Bromelain: Bromelain is an enzyme extracted from pineapples. It is responsible for breaking down proteins. A review of the scientific literature has shown bromelain to protect against cancer, have anti-inflammatory properties, enhance wound healing and enhance circulatory and cardiovascular health.[69,70] Therapeutic effects can be achieved with higher doses.

Papain: Papain is an enzyme that is extracted from the papaya plant. It breaks down protein as well as meat fibers. A review of the scientific literature pertaining to papain has shown it to have tremendous benefits in wound healing.

Pepsin: Pepsin is a key player in digesting protein and as compared to its plant enzyme counterparts (bromelain or papain) it has more active anti-bacterial activity.[71] When it breaks down proteins, the by-products that are produced can decrease gram-negative bacteria that can aggravate the digestive tract and contribute to SIBO.

Amylase: Amylase is produced in human saliva and is responsible for breaking down carbohydrates. Amylase is also produced by the pancreas and is excreted into the small intestine for digestion. There is still a lot of research that needs to be done, but some preliminary research speculates that the gene responsible for producing amylase plays a role in one's risk of developing diseases like diabetes.[72]

Lipase: Lipase is responsible for breaking down fat as well as mobilizing fat from fat stores. If you cannot break fat down properly, energy metabolism is affected negatively and this can contribute to obesity and insulin resistance.

Cellulase: Cellulase is produced by the fermentation of bacteria that naturally occur in the large intestine. It is responsible for breaking down fibrous plants, specifically the cellulose found in plants. The large intestine does not produce enough cellulase, and therefore a lot of cellulose is excreted in the feces. A cellulase supplement can help to maintain a balanced blood sugar level, as cellulase decreases the absorption of glucose (sugar). An increase in cellulase also allows you to benefit from the nutrition that many fibrous plants have to offer.

Invertase: Invertase is an enzyme that is made by bees (found in pollen) or is found in baker's yeast. It is responsible for breaking down sucrose into fructose and glucose. Systemically, it can help to boost the immune system, can increase metabolism and has antioxidant and antimicrobial properties.

The above enzymes can be found naturally in raw foods. However, if we are trying to heal the gut, we need to cook fruits and vegetables in order to give the gut a chance to heal. Some raw foods that you can include in your gut-healing regimen, however, are the following:

- Raw honey
- Bee pollen
- Raw dairy (if tolerated)
- Extra virgin olive oil
- Extra virgin coconut oil
- Avocado

Once your gut is healed, you can also include the following foods:

- Papaya (if tolerated)
- Pineapple
- Mango (if tolerated)
- Kiwi
- Grapes

(I always say, "if tolerated," because some of the foods I mention here can cause autoimmune attacks in certain individuals).

In my experience, however, I generally recommend an enzyme supplement in order to help with digestion. Things to look out for specifically when buying an enzyme supplement include the following:

- Make sure that there are multiple enzymes included (like the ones mentioned previously).
- Look for the enzymatic activity of each enzyme, not just weight
- As with all supplements, make sure natural ingredients are used with no additives and that the supplements come from a reputable source that engages in third-party lab testing to ensure that you are actually getting what you paid for.

Again, work with a health care practitioner in order to find out which and how many enzymes work for you.

Ox Bile

An unhealthy gut can also lead to inefficient bile production. This could lead to gall bladder and liver toxicity and interfere with proper digestion of fats. In fact, people with impaired gut function can find excess undigested fat in their feces because of this. (This is called steatorrhea.)

One study where part of the small intestine was removed in a patient with Crohn's disease, showed that taking exogenous ox bile helped to alleviate steatorrhea (undigested fat in the feces).[77]

If you notice an oily stool or you have stools that float, this may be a sign that you are not absorbing fat properly. An ox bile supplement can help to alleviate this issue. Ask your doctor if it is appropriate for you.

Probiotics

A balance between good and bad bacteria is vital to proper gut health. If there are not enough good bacteria in the gut, the gut and ultimately overall health are compromised.

A meta-analysis on the effects of probiotics on irritable bowel syndrome showed that patients who took probiotics, saw an improvement in their symptoms, as compared to those who took a placebo.[78] This is a very good sign that probiotics contribute to healing the gut.

Foods with Naturally Occurring Probiotics:

Sauerkraut or kimchi.

Sauerkraut and kimchi are basically fermented cabbage. These are a cheap and very easy way of obtaining probiotics, whose count in these foods could easily reach one trillion. Probiotics found in fermented Chinese cabbage were found to reduce cholesterol levels in mice, therefore suggesting that it does contain live bacteria.

Kambucha.

Kambucha is a fermented beverage made from tea and bacteria cultures. It has been used for thousands of years to stimulate the metabolism and to support a healthy immune system. Making it at home is easy and cheap.

Kefir and yogurt.

Kefir and yogurt are both forms of fermented milk products. Again, not all people can tolerate dairy products and in general, goat's milk and sheep's milk are more easily digested than cow's milk.

Coconut or water kefir.

If you cannot tolerate dairy products, you can make kefir from water or coconut milk. You would need to purchase kefir grains to do this.

Including any of the listed foods into a daily meal plan will greatly increase the beneficial bacteria in your intestine and this will result in better health and overall well-being.

If you choose a probiotic to take as a supplement, it is important to consider the strains that are used and how much of each are used. In general, many different strains of probiotics in the billion range per capsule are recommended in order to supplement an unhealthy gut. It is prudent to mention that one should start with a lower dose and work their way up to avoid uncomfortable gas and bloating symptoms.

Following is a chart of probiotic strains to look for:

Bacillus subtilis	*Lactobacillus brevis*	*Lactobacillus lactis*
Bifidobacterium bifidum	*Lactobacillus bilgaricus*	*Lactobacillus plantarum*
Bifidobacterium breve	*Lactobacillus casei*	*Lactobacillus reuteri*
Bifidobacterium infantis	*Lactobacillus delbruecki*	*Lactobacillus rhamnosus*
Bifidobacterium longum	*Lactobacillus DDS-1*	*Lactobacillus salivarius*
Lactobacillus acidophilus	*Lactobacillus helveticus*	*Streptococcus thermophilus*

To give an example of how different strains work, *Bifidobacterium bifidum* is an anaerobe bacteria (this means it can survive without oxygen) that has been shown by studies to decrease the effect of diarrhea caused by rotavirus on the gut.[80]

Lactobacillus casei has been found to modulate the composition and metabolic activity of the intestinal flora.[81]

Other considerations for choosing a probiotic:

- **Can it survive stomach acid**? By using a probiotic we want to inoculate the small intestine. However, if the coating of the probiotic is not acid resistant, a lot of the beneficial bacteria will not reach the small intestine. Manufacturers use enteric coatings for this purpose, but there is not sufficient research to know if these enteric coatings are effective and how many beneficial bacteria actually reach the gut.

  One method you can try is to open the probiotic capsule and dilute it in water. Then take this mixture on an empty stomach. The stomach takes only fifteen to twenty minutes to empty liquid, and therefore the transit time through the stomach and its harsh acid is lowered, giving the probiotics more opportunity to make it to the small intestine.

- **Time kills.** Remember that probiotics are living organisms, and therefore the longer they are living on a shelf, the greater the chance that you are not getting a viable product. Always check the packaging date of the probiotics to get an idea of their shelf-life. Also, once they are opened, keep probiotics refrigerated to protect them against further damage.

Glutamine.

Glutamine is an amino acid that is vital to the health of the intestine. In hospitals, it has been shown to prevent the deterioration of the gut as well as to preserve its integrity.[84] This has been known for a while, as I remember in my dietetic internship always including a glutamine supplement into the patient's regimen when gut integrity was impaired. There is also some research that shows that glutamine can restore immune function which is great news for people with Hashimoto's disease.[85] Glutamine is also a vital amino acid associated with phase 2 detoxification in the liver. Glutamine supplementation is warranted when trying to repair a leaky gut.

Coenzyme Q10.

Coenzyme Q10 is part of every cell in the body and is used to produce energy. It also acts as an antioxidant that helps fight free radicals. As we age, our capacity to produce coenzyme Q10 diminishes.

Coenzyme Q10 is also important for gut health. In a 2016 animal study, the administration of coenzyme Q10, in addition to medication, was found to protect against ulcerative colitis better than medication alone.[86]

Zinc.

Zinc is a mineral whose level is typically low in people who are hypothyroid. Supplementation with zinc has been shown to decrease intestinal permeability.

N-acetyl cysteine.

N-acetyl cysteine is a precursor to glutathione which is the body's ultimate antioxidant and is needed by the liver to detoxify the body. Glutathione levels are also low in hypothyroid patients, and it is not well absorbed if taken orally. N-acetyl cysteine has been shown to boost glutathione production and decrease intestinal permeability.

Healing the gut takes time and commitment. Use this chapter as a guideline to asking questions of your health care practitioner in order to optimize your healing process.

CHAPTER 3

THE SYSTEM TRIO AND YOUR THYROID

Immune System Support

The immune system is an intricate web of processes that happen within the body to help us combat deleterious foreign invaders. This is a system that is vital for our survival. However, sometimes the immune system begins to work against us. One example of this is Hashimoto's thyroiditis. In order to understand how the immune system contributes to or falters when one has Hashimoto's thyroiditis, it is important to learn about some of the different aspects that are involved. Since Hashimoto's is, in essence, a disease of the immune system that attacks the thyroid, learning nutritional tactics to balance the immune system is crucial to healing.

Parts of the immune system involved in the autoimmune response

TH1 Pathway

TH1 cells are part of the immune system and are involved in what is called cell-mediated immunity. They fight off pathogens that exist inside of the cell, specifically viruses, fungi, protozoans, cancers and bacteria. The TH1 pathway does not produce antibodies. It activates phagocytes, natural killer cells and antigen-specific cytotoxic T-lymphocytes that kill viruses.

This part of the immune system is pro-inflammatory (or causes inflammation which is responsible for causing symptoms such as muscle and joint pain, headaches, etc.) and is associated with IG2 antibodies like the ones seen in Hashimoto's. Most people with Hashimoto's thyroiditis are TH1 dominant. This means that the TH1 pathway is over-active and causes an imbalance of the immune system. Once this imbalance occurs, the immune system is capable of attacking healthy tissue, such as seen with Hashimoto's thyroiditis.

TH2 Pathway

This pathway is known as the humoral-mediated pathway, which literally means that it is associated with the substances found outside of the cells in body fluids. Cytokines produced in this pathway fight off parasites that exist between the cells and decrease the TH1 pro-inflammatory response. Instead, B cells are created, which are antibodies that mark the invaders and lead the immune response. The TH2 pathway is associated with the IgE mediated response, which is responsible for seasonal allergies as well as anaphylactic shock.

TH17

TH17 produces pro-inflammatory cytokines against microbes such as *Citrobacter, Klebsiella pneumonia* and *Candida albicans* and can start an autoimmune reaction. TH17 is associated with both Hashimoto's and Grave's disease.

T Regulatory Cells

T regulatory cells (Tregs) are responsible for bringing the body back to balance after an infection. They are anti-inflammatory and immunosuppressive and promote immune system tolerance (against autoimmunity). There is an inverse relationship between Tregs and TH17. An increase of TH17 can decrease Tregs. Low amounts of Tregs are seen in Hashimoto's.

A Protocol for Immune System Support

We would be negligent to not address how we can improve immune function in order to alleviate a lot of the symptoms associated with Hashimoto's disease. The following is a protocol that is given by a pioneer in thyroid disease support, Dr. Datis Kharrazian. He outlines what needs to be done in order to support the immune system:

1. **Support the T-regulatory cells:** In people with Hashimoto's, people typically have lowered levels of T-regulatory cells, causing the immune system to dysfunction and attack healthy tissue like, that in the thyroid gland. In order to support the proper functioning of T-regulatory cells, it is important to give therapeutic doses of vitamin D. Dr. Kharrazian states that, "studies have found that more than 90 percent of people with autoimmune thyroid disease have a genetic defect affecting their ability to process vitamin D. Therefore, they need higher amounts of vitamin D to maintain health."

Glutathione and superoxide dismutase are also powerful antioxidants that help to support the immune system. (These antioxidants are more effective when absorbed through the skin). Fish oil is also very effective at supporting the immune system.

2. **Balance TH-1 and TH-2**: With autoimmune disease, one part of the immune system could be working harder than the other. The TH-1 side is made up of natural killer and cytotoxic T-cells, whereas the TH-2 side is made up of B-cell antibodies. If you are TH-1 dominant, you can stimulate the TH-2 side so that both sides of the immune system become balanced. Likewise, if you are TH-2 dominant, you can stimulate the TH-1 side. Things like coffee, green tea, and grape seed extract can increase TH-2 if TH-1 is dominant, and things like Echinacea and Glycyrrhiz can increase TH-1 if TH-2 is dominant. Elevated TH-1 or TH-2 cytokines block thyroid receptor sites, making it harder for cells to use T3 hormones for metabolism.

    Compounds that modulate both TH-1 and TH-2 and dampen the activation of both include probiotics, vitamin A and E, colostrum, *Boswellia*, pancreatic enzymes and turmeric/curcumin.

3. **Remove the antigen.** In the case of Hashimoto's, the most common antigen that can trigger an autoimmune attack on the thyroid is gluten. Simply excluding gluten-containing

products from the diet can put the immune attack into remission.

Please note that the above is a very simplified version of how to manage an autoimmune disease like Hashimoto's. For more detailed information, I highly recommend you read Dr. Kharrazian's book, *Why Do I Still Have Thyroid Symptoms, When My Lab Tests Are Normal?* Also, take a look at *Hashimoto's Thyroiditis, Lifestyle Interventions for Finding and Treating the Root Cause* by Izabella Wentz.

It is vital to address supporting the immune system along with the thyroid when trying to heal thyroid disease.

Nutritional Support for the Immune System

In a study performed in the *International Journal of Celiac Disease* that aimed to calculate the percentage increase of autoimmune disease worldwide, the authors stated that there is a recognizable trend that attributes the rise in autoimmune incidence to environmental factors rather than genetic factors.[3]

Nutrition is a *huge* environmental factor that we *can* control in order to prevent and heal disease. In this case, there are many nutritional factors that can help balance and optimize immune function so that the immune system supports the body instead of attacking it.

The following are important nutrients to consider when trying to balance the immune system.

Vitamin D3

The importance of vitamin D to the immune system cannot be emphasized enough. There is a myriad of recent research showing that vitamin D can help protect against cancer, cardiovascular disease, diabetes, neurologic disease and specifically autoimmune disease.[4]

Vitamin D3 is made in the skin as a direct response to ultraviolet rays from sunlight. The classic pathway of vitamin D3 is that it is made into the active form by the liver and then helps calcium to be absorbed. However, research now shows that immune system cells also have vitamin D receptors and use it for many different purposes. In fact, vitamin D is able to alter innate immunity (the immune system one is born with) as well as adaptive immunity (how the immune system changes in response to environmental triggers).

To give just one example, macrophages (white blood cells) produce the anti-bacterial peptide LL-37 in response to endogenously produced vitamin D to enhance innate immunity.[5] In other words, the immune system is boosted with sufficient levels of vitamin D in the blood.

A study done at Pennsylvania State University in 2004 suggested that vitamin D does, in fact, play a role in decreasing the incidence and severity of autoimmune diseases.[6] In other words, proper levels of vitamin D can help to prevent and to put certain autoimmune conditions into remission.

In the case of an autoimmune disease such as Hashimoto's thyroiditis, vitamin D helps to balance the immune system by enhancing the effect of T-lymphocytes.

As mentioned earlier, there is evidence that people with Hashimoto's are not able to process vitamin D as well as those without an autoimmune disorder, and therefore a normal-high level of vitamin D in the blood is recommended. It is important to note, however, that this is also dependant on proper vitamin A and K2 concentration. If these two vitamins are deficient, a high serum vitamin D level may be toxic. Dosage depends on the individual, and therefore working with a clinician who knows about vitamin D is essential when taking supplements.

How much sunlight does a person need?

The most effective way to get adequate amounts of vitamin D is through sun exposure. One study showed that a moment of ultraviolet radiation from a sunbed was equivalent to taking up to 25,000 IU of vitamin D3 from supplements.[7]

So, how much sunlight do you need? It is difficult to answer this question as vitamin D3 production varies due to skin pigmentation, where a person lives, season and time of day. If a person knows that after thirty minutes of sun exposure he or she will get a mild sunburn, then exposure of the face, arms, and legs for 20 to 25 percent of that time (six to eight minutes) two to three times a week is enough to prevent vitamin D deficiency.

In the absence of direct sunlight, 800 to 1,000 IU of vitamin D3 supplementation per day is needed to prevent vitamin D deficiency.

According to Dr. Holick, an expert in vitamin D supplementation and author of the book, *The Vitamin D Solution*, it is safe to ingest up to 5,000 to 6,000 IU of vitamin D3 for two to three months in the presence of a vitamin D deficiency. Of course, it goes without saying that this should be done under the supervision of a doctor.

Omega-3 Fatty Acids

Omega-3 fatty acids decrease inflammation and thus have a positive influence in balancing the immune system. Many studies have confirmed the benefits of dietary supplementation in autoimmune diseases like lupus, Crohn's disease, and ulcerative colitis.

Many of the placebo-controlled trials of fish oil in chronic inflammatory diseases have revealed significant benefits, including decreased disease activity and a lowered use of anti-inflammatory drugs.[9]

More specific information on which foods contain omega-3 fatty acids and which supplements to take will be provided later in this book.

Probiotics

As previously mentioned in chapter two, the microbiome can be described as all the bacteria, parasites, and viruses that we are host to. Just as the earth is the host to all of us humans, we are host to tiny creatures that can either support or destroy our health.

There is research to suggest that the delicate balance of good versus bad bacteria in the body can affect the immune system.

A study done at the Kingston General Hospital in Kingston, Ontario in March 2016 found that the microbiome of people with irritable bowel syndrome was changed after a three-week low FODMAPs diet was implemented. Seventy-two percent of patients with IBS saw a fifty-percent or greater reduction in symptoms on this diet.[10] (This type of diet will be explored in more detail later). This study basically showed that optimizing the microbiome via diet, reduced the symptoms of IBS. This is very exciting as we see proof that the diet can change the types of bacteria that live within us and that ultimately affect our immune system!

Another recent study linked the microbiome to decreasing the chances of autoimmune disease and diabetes. Researchers have found that antimicrobial peptides called CRAMP (cathelicidins) decrease the incidence of diabetes and autoimmune disease. When CRAMP was administered to pre-diabetic mice (non-obese pre-diabetic), it regulated the immune cells in the pancreatic islets, dampening the incidence of autoimmune diabetes. The study also showed that short chain fatty acids produced by the microbiota play a vital role in regulating CRAMP and therefore can have a profound effect on the development of autoimmune disease.[11]

The above studies are a few of the many examples that demonstrate a link between our microbiota, diet, and autoimmune disease.

Most of us need a reinoculation of good bacteria or probiotics to help ensure a healthy and balanced microbiome. Such a reinoculation can help to enhance the immune system and ultimately put an autoimmune attack into remission.

A recent randomized, double-blind, placebo-controlled study described in the *Journal of Clinical Gastroenterology* showed that in Celiac disease patients who did *not* follow a gluten-free diet who were given the probiotic *B.infantis,* although there was no change in intestinal permeability, there were significant improvements in gastrointestinal symptoms as well as a decrease in TG2 and IgA antibodies. This study provided further proof of the fact that the microbiota can influence an autoimmune response.[12]

For more specific recommendations on probiotics, refer to chapter two.

Vitamin A

In a Venezualan study, Jimenez et al. tested the effect of a single dose of 200,000 IU of vitamin A on iron status, nutritional status of vitamin A, and the phagocytic function of neutrophils in preschool children. The follow-up one month after giving the vitamin A showed a decrease in anemia and an increase in phagocytic capacity in the children who received the vitamin A supplementation. This study showed promise as to how vitamin A can enhance immune system function.[13]

It is important to know that vitamin A status is highly dependant on zinc and iron status. Zinc is responsible for the synthesis of the protein that vitamin A binds to in order to be transferred to peripheral tissues. If there isn't enough zinc to create this protein, there is a good chance that one will be deficient in of vitamin A.

Randomized double-blind placebo studies have found that vitamin A deficiency cannot be alleviated with vitamin A supplementation in the presence of an iron deficiency.[14] The exact method by which iron affects vitamin A metabolism is not known at this time.

This interaction between vitamin A, zinc, and iron is one of the many examples of how vitamins and minerals work together to preserve the metabolism and the immune system of the human body. It is very important to remember that a single deficiency can cause a cascade of symptoms due to the fact that vitamins and minerals work synergistically in the body.

Vitamin E

Vitamin E is a very powerful antioxidant. There are eight types of vitamin E: alpha, beta, gamma, delta tocopherol and alpha, beta, gamma, delta tocotrienol. All are important and each serves a different function within the body.

After Evans and Bishop, in 1922, discovered that dietary supplements of alfalfa leaves (which are rich in vitamin E) could prevent placental hemorrhage and reverse dietary sterility in rats, vitamin E was given its name. It comes from the Greek words, tocos (child birth), *pheros* (to bear),and ol (alcohol).

The tocopherols are lipophilic, or attracted to fat, where-as the tocotrienols are unsaturated and able to penetrate into tissues that have saturated fatty layers, such as the brain and the liver. A review of tocotrienols in 2014 showed that tocotrienols may be superior to the tocopherols for disease prevention. They have antioxidant and anti-inflammatory effects and have neuroprotective, cholesterol-lowering, and anticancer properties.[15]

Tocotrienols are found predominantly in foods such as palm oil, rice bran oil, coconut oil, barley germ, wheat germ, and annatto. Palm oil and rice bran oil contain the most tocotrienols (940mg/kg and 465 mg/kg, respectively).[16]

The fact that vitamin E has been shown to have many anti-inflammatory effects within the body shows its promise for boosting immune health and ultimately reducing autoimmune symptoms.

Boswelia

A review of the literature regarding the use of herbs to treat ulcerative colitis (an autoimmune disorder of the gut) showed that *Boswelia* was more effective than the placebo in putting ulcerative colitis into remission. The authors of the review suggested that more research is needed to give more conclusive recommendations, however, the literature does suggest that *Boswe lia* could have a positive effect in decreasing autoimmune symptoms.[19]

Curcumin

Curcumin is a substance found in the spice turmeric. Several studies have found curcumin to help with pro-inflammatory diseases such as cancer, arthritis, IBS, and Crohn's disease. It has the ability to modulate specific cytokines of the immune system as well as detoxification agents such as glutathione. Since it has this quality, curcumin has a big effect on how the immune system works.

A study done on patients with ulcerative colitis and Crohn's disease, showed a decrease in symptoms with curcumin supplementation.[20] Although more large-scale, double-blind and placebo-controlled studies are needed to confirm the use of curcumin in autoimmune diseases such as ulcerative colitis, many studies such as this showed promise for the use of curcumin to decrease symptoms.

The literature shows that up to eight grams per day of curcumin can be used safely to enhance its therapeutic effects.

Antioxidant-Rich Foods

Antioxidants are basically scavengers that seek and destroy free radicals. Free radicals created from things like environmental toxins, processed foods, or smoking cause damage to healthy cells and tissues, thus hindering the immune system from working properly.

Antioxidants are found in fruits and vegetables, especially in foods such as berries, nuts and seeds, and green leafy vegetables such as kale and spinach. The phytochemicals found in these foods have anti-inflammatory effects and should definitely be included in a protocol to balance the immune system.

A double-blind, randomize, and placebo-controlled study published in the *European Journal of Clinical Nutrition* found that sea buckthorn berries were able to decrease levels of C-reactive protein (CRP), a marker of inflammation.[21]

What Foods Can Cause an Autoimmune Flare-Up?

Just as important as adding specific nutrients to the diet to help balance the immune system is removing foods from the diet that are known to cause inflammation and fuel an autoimmune attack. As stated previously, gluten found in foods like wheat, barley, and rye is one such trigger.

The obvious example of a gluten intolerance can be seen with Celiac disease. However, further research has shown us that a gluten-free diet can alter the microbiome, which can decrease the rate of pro-inflammatory cytokines released by the bacteria found in the intestine.

In a study published by the *British Journal of Nutrition*, a gluten-free diet was found to decrease an immune response by decreasing the production of pro-inflammatory cytokines by gut bacteria.[22]

Studies such as these show that environmental factors, such as removing gluten from the diet, can prevent the immune system from attacking otherwise healthy tissue.

What about Dairy?

For many, dairy products, especially those produced by conventional farming, can also cause inflammation.

In my experience, when I give patients an anti-inflammatory protocol, I typically remove gluten-containing foods along with dairy. Once improvement in symptoms is seen, I may reintroduce organic versions of dairy, but I am more strict on sticking to a gluten-free lifestyle.

Nutrition can definitely play a role in balancing the immune system in order to alleviate symptoms associated with autoimmune disorders. If you do not get enough organic, wild-caught fatty fish in your diet, it's a good idea to start supplementing with omega-3 fatty acids. Adding curcumin to your supplement protocol is also a good idea. Definitely keep track of your vitamin D status. If you cannot get enough time in the sun, work with your doctor to make sure you are taking the right supplements.

In terms of diet, omit gluten from your daily meal plan. If you do not want to cut dairy, choose organic, grass-fed dairy from local farmers. In general, grass-fed dairy has a higher nutrient density in the form of vitamins A and E, omega-3 fatty acids, and vitamin D (all of which help support the immune system).

Also, a great way to incorporate antioxidant-rich foods into your diet is to include daily smoothies. Make smoothies with berries, kale and other fruits and vegetables that you enjoy in order to make sure you get their immune-boosting effects.

Case Study

A thirty-five year old female with a long history of IBS and constipation came to me as she was diagnosed with Hashimoto's thyroiditis. She wanted to see if nutrition could help to relieve her symptoms. She complained about feeling so sleepy throughout the day that she could not concentrate at work and would fall asleep without realizing it. She had also gained weight and could not lose it with traditional dieting tactics. She was depressed.

I put her on an anti-inflammatory and low-residue diet (as she claimed that anything raw would bother her). I excluded gluten and dairy from her diet and recommended bone broth, a collagen supplement and a prescription of supplements that included omega 3 fatty acids, vitamin D3, vitamin K2, probiotics, vitamin B complex, curcumin and an antioxidant rich vitamin.

After only one month, her energy came back, she could concentrate, she started to lose weight and according to her, she felt that she had been brought back to life.

She now adamantly stays away from grains, she is able to tolerate some fermented dairy, she eats raw vegetables and salads and has adapted a new eating pattern in order to maintain her new-found health.

This definitely was a success story for me as a health practitioner because in this case, diet was the key to offering someone a better quality of life.

A Common Sense Approach to Supporting Adrenal Health

My great-grandfather lived in a village on the Mediterranean island of Cyprus all his life. He never went to the doctor, he ate organic food off of his land he got plenty of sunshine and exercise, he enjoyed his family (he had eighteen children!), and he died at the age of ninety-three because he fell while he was climbing a tree. I don't know about you, but most modern-day twenty year-olds have a hard time getting to the gym, let alone have the physical skills to climb a tree!

The point of all of this is to compare some lifestyles of the past to our modern-day way of life and to point out the tremendous role that emotional and physical stress play in our hormonal health.

Today, instead of living off the land we depend on the food industry to feed us (a fact that has taught many of us to depend on processed foods). We have sedentary lifestyles, we barely connect with nature, we are switched on to marketing messages and social media throughout the day, we are stressed out because we are trying to find ways to pay the bills instead of connecting with our families, we pop pills to ignore our body's natural warning signals just to get through the day, we don't get enough rest, we have trouble sleeping and the list goes on and on.

I think you get the picture. All the above can wreak havoc on your thyroid because your adrenal glands, which are walnut-shaped organs that sit on top of the kidneys, are constantly in a state of panic, producing stress hormones such as cortisol, epinephrine, and norepinephrine that allow us to deal with the heavy emotional and physical load most of us endure on a daily basis.

The stress response is a great way for the body to cope in times of hardship. Imagine that it is an alarm bell that sounds to warn the rest of the body that there is danger. It sends a signal for the body to stop unnecessary processes for short periods of time in order to deal with the danger and then move on. Imagine you are about to be attacked by a bear. Your body will pump out stress hormones to slow your digestion and increase your awareness so that you can run for your life.

Now imagine that this stress response is happening all day, every day. This is definitely a recipe for disaster, as your body operates at a suboptimal rate when it is always in a state of panic.

The symptoms of adrenal fatigue are very similar to those of hypothyroidism. In fact, many people who think they are dealing with a thyroid problem may not have a thyroid problem at all. The root cause of all their symptoms may simply be overworked adrenal glands. Therefore, if you suspect a thyroid problem, it is crucial that you also check your adrenal function in order to rule out an underlying issue.

The symptoms of adrenal fatigue are as follows:

- Fatigue
- Headaches
- Decreased immunity
- Difficulty falling asleep or staying asleep and waking up
- Mood swings
- Sugar and caffeine cravings
- Irritability or light-headedness between meals
- Eating to relieve fatigue
- Dizziness when moving from sitting or lying to standing
- Gastric ulcers

The Adrenal Glands and Thyroid Function

There are several ways that the adrenal glands can affect thyroid function: [23]

1. **HPA axis disruption**

   The adrenal glands work hand in hand with the hypothalamus and pituitary glands to control hormonal balance. As previously discussed, the pituitary gland is responsible for signalling the thyroid to produce thyroid hormones. Therefore, if the adrenal glands do not send the proper signals to the hypothalamus and pituitary glands, thyroid function will be suppressed.

A preliminary study done in 2012 on healthy men and women with subclinical hypothyroidism (elevated TSH but normal free T3 and free T4) showed that there was a direct correlation between cortisol and TSH hormone. This suggests that if there is adrenal fatigue or if too much cortisol is produced, it throws off the balance of the thyroid.[24]

Inflammatory cytokines released during the stress response are responsible for throwing off the HPA axis and suppressing thyroid function.

2. **Reduction in conversion from T4 to T3**

The same inflammatory cytokines that suppress thyroid function through the HPA axis are also responsible for decreasing the conversion from inactive thyroid hormone, T4, to the active thyroid hormone, T3.

3. **Increased risk of autoimmunity**

Adrenal stress weakens barriers within the body (in the intestines, lungs and brain) that protect the rest of the body from foreign invaders. Therefore, antigens, bacteria and proteins that are not supposed to enter the bloodstream do, and this throws the immune system out of balance. When this happens, there is a higher likelihood of autoimmune disease.

4. **Thyroid hormone resistance**

Cytokines released during periods of stress are also responsible for decreasing thyroid hormone sensitivity. This is why a lot of people with normal thyroid labs on medication can see no improvement in symptoms. There may be enough hormones, but the cells simply do not use the hormone for metabolic functioning.

5. **Hormonal imbalance in general**

When your body does not clear estrogen properly, a build-up of estrogen results that increases thyroid binding globules (TBG). TBG is responsible for carrying T4 and T3 around in the blood. If these thyroid hormones are not "free" from their carriers (TBG), they cannot enter the cells to do their work. Stress hormones like cortisol decrease the liver's ability to clear excess estrogen from the body, and therefore decrease the amount of free thyroid hormone available for use by the cells.

A Common Sense Approach to Balancing Your Adrenals.

As my parents have been saying for years, "Unfortunately, common sense is not so common anymore." I find that we take factors that should be common knowledge for most of us for granted and do not consider them when trying to improve our health. What do I mean? Factors like sleep, staying well hydrated, not drinking too much coffee, decreasing stress and the like, we often put on the backburner and do not take as serious players when it comes to chronic afflictions. Yet, these lifestyle factors, when ignored, can have serious consequences on our health.

Circadian Rhythms – The Rhythm Is Gonna Get You!

As we are inhabitants of the earth, we are also sensitive to the earth's natural rhythms. All of us are programmed internally to respond to what is going on around us at specific times of the day. Sunlight and darkness signal specific hormones to work in order to wake us up and put us to sleep, respectively. Even thyroid hormones have a circadian rhythm. According to Dr. Alan Christiansen, a naturopathic medical doctor that specializes in holistic therapies for issues like adrenal health, T3 is produced in the middle of the night as we sleep. Therefore, taking thyroid medication before we sleep or as soon as we wake up is the ideal way to mimic the body's natural production of T3.

Stress hormones like cortisol, should be high in the morning (helping us to wake up) and low at night (allowing us to calm down and sleep). Factors such as poor sleeping habits, poor diet, having bright lights on at night, staring at television or lap top screens at night, too much coffee intake and stress can all affect this delicate circadian rhythm. People who do not go to sleep until 1:00 am and wake up at 7:00 am throw off their cortisol rhythm and therefore have increased chances of blood glucose imbalances, excess fat around the midsection and weight gain in general.

How Does Cortisol Affect Blood Sugar?

Blood sugar levels should optimally be between 80 and 110 in the blood. Even fluctuating between these numbers too many times throughout the day could cause problems. Cortisol responds to low blood glucose concentration in the blood. For example, if you have gone many hours without eating, cortisol is responsible for making glucose out of glycogen stores in the liver and muscles (you can think of glycogen as the short-term glucose reserve formed from eating carbohydrates) in order to increase blood sugar levels. If you do not eat enough carbohydrates, however, cortisol still provides glucose, but it does it by breaking down muscle tissue.

Now imagine that your cortisol levels are completely out of whack. For example, if you do not produce enough cortisol because you have adrenal dysregulation, when you go for a while without eating, you get irritable, shaky, and perhaps even dizzy, as there is not enough cortisol in your body to pull your blood sugar back up to normal.

We need cortisol to maintain our blood sugar levels, and we can help to maintain proper cortisol levels by eating in a way that supports its natural production within the body.

How Cortisol Dysregulation Makes Us Gain Weight

Cortisol and blood glucose imbalance can be the cause of weight gain in many people. The simple explanation here is that if there is any dysregulation within the body's natural processes, metabolism is affected. What this means is that if you have an issue with cortisol production, the metabolism goes into hibernation mode and does not use glucose for energy, but instead stores it as fat.

There are more receptors for cortisol in the abdominal area than in any other area of the body, and since consistently high cortisol levels increase fat in the midsection, it is no wonder that chronically stressed out people carry their fat in their waist.

There have been studies that link high cortisol levels with higher calorie, simple carbohydrate, and fat intake. In other words, if you are constantly stressed out, you will have more of a tendency to reach for comfort food than when you are not. And of course, eating more processed foods leads to weight gain.

Cortisol decreases the insulin response. Therefore, if cortisol always tries to boost your blood sugar and your cells do not accept the sugar in order to produce energy because of low insulin levels, the extra glucose needs to go somewhere and is therefore stored as fat.

How Do We Regulate Cortisol Levels If We Have Adrenal Fatigue?

The importance of sleep.

One of the best ways the body can recuperate from stress is to sleep. During sleep, the body maintains itself by repairing what needs to be repaired. This includes balancing the immune system, regulating hormonal function and enhancing brain activity. If you do not get enough sleep, cortisol levels are thrown off and a vicious cycle begins.

The ideal time to go to bed is around 10:00 pm. This will give you enough time to wind down before you actually sleep. This is the time of day when cortisol is at its lowest and melatonin (our sleep hormone) is at its highest. If you stay up until midnight, your body considers this a stressful situation and produces more cortisol. This is why a lot of people feel tired around 9:00 pm and can't keep their eyes open, but if they force themselves to stay up, they have trouble falling asleep around 1:00 am. Having a consistent bedtime therefore is imperative in order to regulate adrenal function.

Bedtime rituals.

Just as important as *when* you go to bed is *what you do* before bedtime. Our bodies respond to the sun going down, and therefore bright lights, loud noises and staring at a tv or lap top, are things that are *not* conducive to helping your body to wind down. So, here are some tips for what to do before bedtime:

1. Try to avoid working on your lap top late at night. If this is not possible, there are special programs you can download that allow your lap-top to know when it is night and reduces screen power for night-time viewing.

2. Many of us *love* to watch television at night, and for many of us it is a way of winding down. However, it can affect our sleep patterns in a negative way. Try to shut off the television one hour before sleep and do some other activity that will prepare you for sleep, like taking a bath, reading, breathing deeply, meditating, or praying.

3. Make sure you take the time to wind down before sleep. Going for a five-mile run before bedtime, for example, is usually not a good idea.

Foods that can promote sleep.

There are a number of foods that can help to promote sleep if incorporated into a daily meal plan.

Maca.

Maca is a tube root that is grown in areas of the world like China. Research shows that it enhances fertility, reduces blood glucose levels and blood pressure, improves memory, reduces anxiety and depression, fights fatigue and is an antioxidant and anti-aging agent.

A number of the components found in Maca, including hexadecanoic acid in fatty acids, calcium and potassium, help to promote sleep.[25]

Panax ginseng.

Asian ginseng has a history of use going back as far as five thousand years. It is known to fight viral infections, reduce stress, boost memory, lower blood sugar and cholesterol and have anti-aging properties.

With regard to sleep, in a study of twenty-two women, Panax

ginseng alleviated menstrual irregularity and pain and also significantly alleviated insomnia, flushing, perspiration and appetite.[26]

Lingzhi.

Otherwise known as *Ganoderma lucidum*, lingzhi has been used as a tranquilizing agent for the treatment of insomnia in China. It has four hundred bioactive compounds, some of which promote sleep.[27]

Increased fruit and vegetable versus confectionary and noodles.

Interestingly enough, research shows that a diet high in sugar and processed white flour not only is deleterious to our overall health but decreases sleep quality as well. In a study looking at sleep duration and diet in teenagers in the *British Journal of Nutrition*, short sleep duration was associated with increased odds of fast-food consumption and less fruit and vegetable consumption.[28]

In another study looking at the eating habits and sleep quality of Japanese workers, a low intake of vegetables and fish and a high intake of confectionary and noodles were independently associated with poor sleep quality.[29]

Other foods that are shown in studies to enhance sleep quality are lettuce, cherries, tart cherry juice, walnuts and kiwi.

Activities that decrease stress.

It goes without saying that it is important to find ways to decrease stress. Try activities such as yoga or meditation, talk through your problems with friends, take long baths, go for a walk in nature, basically, do whatever will help you to forget your troubles and relax.

The best way to balance the adrenals is to get rid of what is causing you to be stressed out in the first place. For most of us, quitting our jobs or changing an annoying family member is not an option, so finding ways to cope becomes very important.

An Adrenal Reset Diet?

According to Dr. Alan Christianson, author of the book *The Adrenal Reset Diet*, we need to eat in a way that supports the natural functioning of our stress hormones, specifically cortisol. This hormone should be at its highest level in the morning and at its lowest level in the evening.

What foods help to boost cortisol in the morning? Protein-rich foods. Therefore, in opposition to what most of us have been told about breakfast, it should consist predominantly of protein-rich foods with few carbohydrates.

When to Eat Carbs for Optimal Cortisol Production.

After 3:00 pm, you can start to include more carbohydrate-rich foods in your diet, with dinner having more carbohydrates than any other meal. Now, don't misunderstand me and think that having a plateful of pasta for dinner is ideal. It's not. I'm simply saying that this meal should have more carbohydrates than your other meals.

What Types of Carbohydrates Should You Include?

With an autoimmune disorder such as Hashimoto's, it is important to stick to the carbohydrates one can tolerate. For example, low-glycemic index fruits such as berries and cherries, starches such as squash or sweet potatoes, and a large variety of vegetables.

Eating in this way will also help to regulate blood sugar levels. This is imperative to healing the adrenal glands. Since hypothyroidism and metabolic syndrome (a condition in which insulin resistance and increased abdominal fat is seen), seem to go hand-in-hand[31], eating in a way that balances blood sugar levels as well as maintains optimal cortisol levels, not only balances the adrenal glands but also optimizes thyroid function.

Is Eating Every Three Hours the Way to Maintain Optimal Blood Glucose Regulation?

When I was doing my internship at Brigham and Women's Hospital and did my rotation at the Joslin Diabetes Center, we were taught to encourage this sector of patients to eat every three hours in order to stabilize their blood sugar levels.

Unfortunately, for people who have adrenal dysregulation, the same holds true. Fasting, or going longer than three to four hours without eating, causes spikes in cortisol and surges in blood sugar. So, in order to keep this under control, it is important to eat something every three hours. What I have found effective with my clients is to mix a source of protein with a source of low-glycemic carbohydrate. For example, an apple with some almonds or chicken with a salad. Eating in this way helps maintain your blood sugar and decreases your chances of exacerbating your adrenal glands further.

Adaptogenic Herbs and Supplements to Consider with Adrenal Fatigue

Adaptogens are herbs that help to balance the adrenal function of the body. They help to balance the hormones that can wreak havoc when out of control in cases of chronic stress. Following are a few adaptogenic herbs that can be considered when trying to heal your adrenal glands. Again, work with your doctor to see which and how much are ideal for you.

Panax Ginseng

Research shows that Panax ginseng enhances the immune system and contributes to blood-glucose regulation and prevention of cancer.[32]

Licorice (**Glycyrrhiza glabra** *and* **G. uralensis**)

Licorice is an adaptogenic herb that increases the amount of cortisol that is available to the tissues.[33] If you have performed a saliva test and know that your morning cortisol levels are low, taking licorice at this time of day may be an option. Be wary of taking licorice at night, as you do not want to raise cortisol levels before bedtime.

Ashwaganda

Ashwaganda is an adaptogenic herb that has been used for thousands of years in Ayurvedic medicine. It has recently gained attention in the Westernized world for its effects in treating stress and anxiety. More large scale studies need to be performed in order to confirm its efficacy, but, in a recent study looking at the effects of stress on weight loss, subjects who were given Ashwaganda had significant improvements in serum cortisol, body weight, and body mass index.[34]

Ashwaganda stabilizes the body's response to stress. Animal studies have found that Ashwaganda may be just as effective in treating anxiety as some medicines used to treat it.[35]

Ashwaganda has also been shown to be an effective adaptogenic herb for thyroid function. Studies have shown that it can increase T4 levels in the blood and it may help stabilize thyroid function in general.[36]

Since Ashwaganda may have a relaxing effect, the ideal time to take it is at night before bedtime.

Holy Basil Leaf

Holy basil leaf is yet another adaptogenic herb that can help with stress. In recent animal studies, holy basil leaf was found to decrease stress by inhibiting the release of cortisol.[37] This is another herb that can be taken in the evening if you know that you have high cortisol levels at night.

Rhodiola

Rhodiola rosea is a traditional Chinese medicine and Scandinavian herb. Scientific literature has shown its effectiveness in relieving fatigue that is caused by stress and burnout. It also is adaptogenic in nature in that it helps to relieve symptoms of stress in people who are fatigued from non-exercise stressors.

There is also some preliminary evidence that rhodiola can decrease stress-induced binge eating in female rats.

Taking a low dose of Rhodiola rosea over a long period of time has been shown to be effective in reducing fatigue caused by stress.[38]

Tyrosine

According to Dr. Shawn Talbott, author of the book T*he Cortisol Connection: Why Stress Makes You Fat and Ruins Your Health*, tyrosine, an amino acid, has been studied as an anti-stress agent. It is a precursor to neurotransmitters such as epinephrine, norepinephrine, and dopamine, all of which are depleted in times of stress, an occurrence that can cause decreases in mental and physical performance. Supplementing with tyrosine has been shown to offset declines in performance that are associated with stress.

Phosphatidylserine (PS)

Phosphatidylserine is a phospholipid found in cells that plays an important role in muscle metabolism and immune function. It has been shown to balance cortisol overproduction, especially following intense exercise. Many athletes use PS to help them recover from intense exercise and to promote muscle growth, as high levels of cortisol break down muscle tissue. Again, if you have high cortisol levels at night, this supplement may also be considered in the evening.

The Adrenals and the Thyroid

If adrenal insufficiency is the root cause of your thyroid problem, implementing some of the suggestions in this chapter will help your thyroid to work optimally. Remember that the adrenal glands and the thyroid work hand in hand so if one is not working properly, chances are the other is not either. I have seen many clients who managed to stay off thyroid medication simply by adapting a lifestyle and meal plan that was conducive to managing stress. If you think faulty adrenals may be your problem, talk with your doctor or functional medicine practitioner to see how you can help yourself.

How Sex Hormones Affect Thyroid Function

If you are beginning to understand the big picture, you are also grasping the fact that the thyroid and its hormones do not work in a vacuum. They collaborate with other hormones. And you guessed it. If these hormones have an imbalance, the thyroid will not function optimally either.

It All Begins with Cholesterol

It's funny how I spent most of my university years learning how to lower cholesterol levels with dietary guidelines. It is ironic that so much research, time and money was invested into how to decrease cholesterol levels to lessen the risk of heart disease, when in fact more focus should have been given to the beneficial aspects of cholesterol. If functional medicine has taught me anything, it is that a multitude of things work together to culminate in disease (or health, for that matter). Cholesterol by itself is not the single predictor of heart disease.

I won't go into the highly controversial debate on whether or not a "high"cholesterol level is good or bad for you. Instead, I will focus on how cholesterol is used by the body to create adrenal and sex hormones.

Cholesterol is used to make pregnenolone, DHEA, progesterone, estrogen, testosterone, and cortisol. Without sufficient cholesterol, there would not be sufficient amounts of sex hormones either. Cholesterol is the single most important precursor to hormonal regulation.

Now let's take a look at each sex hormone and see how it can affect the proper functioning of the thyroid:

Pregnenolone

Pregnenolone is the main precursor to many of our hormones. In times of chronic stress, your body needs to make more cortisol to keep up with the demand for it. When this happens, pregnenolone is "stolen" from other hormones in order to make more cortisol (this is also known as the "pregnenolone steal"). This causes a cascade of hormonal imbalances and deficiencies. You could become deficient in both progesterone and testosterone.

Remember that cortisol imbalances interfere with normal thyroid hormone function, and therefore if you have adrenal dysregulation, supplementing with pregnenolone could help to restore adrenal function, which will, in turn, boost thyroid function.

DHEA

DHEA is created from pregnenolone and is the precursor to testosterone and estrogen. It has key functions in muscle building, tissue repair, immune function, energy production, fat burning and liver function.

Progesterone

Thyroid hormone and progesterone work hand in hand. You need thyroid hormone in order to produce enough progesterone and you need progesterone in order to have optimal thyroid function. Progesterone is increased after day twenty-one of a menstrual cycle and is needed to build the uterine lining during pregnancy. For many, infertility is due to low progesterone levels, which many times can be caused by hypothyroidism (or insufficient amounts of T4 and T3 hormones). Also, in times of stress where pregnenolone is stolen to make cortisol, not enough progesterone *or* thyroid hormones are produced, and this causes a vicious cycle of hormonal imbalance.

Supplements That May Help to Boost Progesterone Production

Chasteberry (*Agnus Castus*).

Agnus castus or chasteberry is an herb that has been traditionally used in Europe to treat female ailments such as premenstrual syndrome and an irregular menstrual cycle. Preliminary research shows that it helps to decrease prolactin levels. This helps to increase progesterone levels allowing for a more regular menstrual cycle.

It should be noted that animal studies have shown that *Agnus castus* can increase TSH and T3, but further research needs to be done in order to ascertain its effect on the thyroid.

Maca.

Maca root is an adaptogenic herb that has been traditionally used to increase sexual libido. Although further studies need to be done to confirm its effects, some research shows that it increases levels of leuteinising hormone, which promotes progesterone production and helps with fertility.

There is limited research on its effects on the thyroid, but some animal studies show that Maca root has no effect on TSH.

Estrogen

Estrogen is a female hormone needed to mature eggs ready for fertilization, and in the right amount it can protect against heart disease and aid in sex drive, brain function and bone health. Unfortunately, however, with the increase of "fake" estrogens in our environment from pesticides, hormones, chemical, and soy additives in our food, estrogen dominance is found in many patients with hormonal imbalance.

Estrogen dominance interferes with the liver's ability to detoxify the body, resulting in toxic amounts of estrogen residues within the body. When this happens, estrogen interferes with proper thyroid hormone functioning in two ways. First, it turns T4 into reverse T3, which is inactive. Second, it binds with the cell receptors that are usually used for thyroid hormones. In other words, if estrogen is attached where T3 comes in to do its work, hypothyroid symptoms could occur because the thyroid hormones cannot get into the cell to produce energy.

Increased stress and adrenal fatigue can also increase levels of inactive estrogens, which can cause moodiness, irritability, and water retention.

Testosterone

Testosterone is also affected by thyroid hormones. When there are not enough thyroid hormones present, testosterone levels also suffer. Interestingly enough, testosterone is just as important for women as it is for men. It is needed for proper libido. If it is too high, it can cause inflammation and acne, and it is common in women with polycystic ovary syndrome. High levels of androgens are also associated with insulin resistance.

Dietary Tactics for Lowering Androgen Levels

High-Fiber, Low-Glycemic Index Diet

If you have constipation issues or digestive issues in general, testosterone is secreted into the bile and then reabsorbed in the gut to be used again. In other words, if you do not eat enough fiber to get rid of excess testosterone, more and more builds up within the body.

Since high testosterone levels are associated with insulin resistance, eating a low-glycemic index diet improves symptoms caused by too many androgens. The glycemic index (GI) is a measure of how many specific carbohydrates raise your blood sugar, on a scale of 100. You should aim for foods that have a GI lower than 55. Studies have found that a low-GI diet decreases insulin-like growth factor, which, in turn decreases acne.

Dairy-Free Diet

Conventional dairy products seem to increase inflammation, which then leads to increased androgen levels and acne. If you remember from previous chapters, dairy is also a common food intolerance that can exacerbate a leaky gut as well as cause an autoimmune attack. Since eating dairy can increase testosterone levels as well, this is just one more reason to exclude it from the diet.

Sugar-Free Diet

It goes without saying that all processed sugars, as well sugar-laden foods, should be taken out of the diet. These foods raise insulin-like growth factor and androgen levels and should be avoided at all costs.

High-Zinc Diet

Zinc deficiency is associated with increased testosterone and acne. To avoid zinc deficiency, eat foods that are naturally high in zinc, such as nuts and seeds, specifically pumpkin and sesame seeds. If nuts and seeds are an issue for you, oysters, as well as red meat and poultry are also high in zinc.

Omega-3 to Omega-6 Balancing Diet

More about the importance of maintaining a good omega-3 to omega-6 balance will be discussed later in this book. However, this is also important when we look at androgens. Women with polycystic ovary syndrome and higher amounts of omega-6 compared to omega-3 have more androgens.[42] Therefore, eating more wild-caught salmon or supplementing with a high-quality omega 3 supplement is also warranted here.

As with any of the above hormones, it is *very* important to find the root cause of why one hormone or another is too high or too low. From my experience as a patient, I tend to opt for trying to find a natural way to balance hormones rather than supplementing with bio-identical hormones. The reason I feel this way is that hormonal regulation is so interconnected that if I were to supplement with one hormone, this might cause a severe imbalance somewhere else. So, *definitely*, work with an integrative doctor whom you trust to see if supplementing with bio-identical hormones is for you.

If you want a great in-depth discussion about hormonal balance, I highly recommend that you read, *The Hormone Cure* by Dr. Sara Gottfried. She is a Harvard-trained integrative, board-certified gynaecologist who finds natural ways of treating hormonal imbalances.

For a better idea about how to eat to balance hormones and to increase fertility (infertility is a not-so-great side effect of having hypothyroidism), I also highly recommend my colleague Vanessa Xenopoulou's book, *Fertility Matters*.

Sex Hormones and the Thyroid

As you can see, thyroid issues can have their root cause in sex hormone imbalance. If you have been on the birth control pill for years, have polycystic ovaries, acne or hair where it shouldn't be, or have trouble sleeping at night, you could have hormonal imbalances. These, in turn, can affect the proper functioning of the thyroid. Therefore, if you suspect that your hormones are out of whack, you may want to explore this further before assuming that your thyroid is at fault. Often, eating clean or doing a cleanse can greatly improve hormonal function and ultimately lead to a healthier thyroid.

CHAPTER 4

FOODS AND ENVIRONMENTAL FACTORS THAT AFFECT THYROID FUNCTION NEGATIVELY

Grains Are Not Your Friend

As mentioned in previous chapters, there is research that shows that gluten is responsible for increased intestinal permeability as well as an increased chance of an autoimmune attack.

In an Italian multicenter study published in the *American Journal of Gastroenterology*, patients with celiac disease who had autoimmune thyroid disease were re-examined after one year on a gluten-free diet. The authors of the study concluded that gluten withdrawal could single-handedly reverse thyroid dysfunction.[1]

Studies such as these allow me to conclude that if you have hypothyroidism, it would be prudent to adopt a gluten-free lifestyle.

What Is Gluten?

Gluten is a family of proteins that is found in foods like wheat, rye, and barley. It is predominantly made up of glutenin and gliadin. When these proteins are mixed with water to create bread, they become sticky and provide a glue that allows the bread to stick together. They are also responsible for making the bread rise, giving bread a fluffy texture.

It is the gliadin part of gluten that is responsible for activating zonulin proteins to increase intestinal permeability. In a study looking specifically at this, gliadin increased intestinal permeability in both celiac and non-celiac (healthy) patients.[2] This could mean that for healthy people, at least limiting the amount of wheat they eat, could decrease possible disease outcomes.

What is Celiac Disease?

Celiac disease is an autoimmune disease in which the immune system attacks gluten proteins as well as the healthy tissue of the lining of the intestine. Celiac disease has major health implications, including digestive issues, anemia and an increased risk of developing other diseases (one of which is autoimmune thyroid disease).[3]

The *only* therapy there is for this disease is the complete exclusion of gluten from the diet. Because this is the case, a lot of research on gluten-free diets focuses on people with celiac disease in order to find a connection between diet and disease progression.

Non-celiac Gluten Sensitivity?

It is estimated that between 0.5 and 13 percent of people have non-celiac gluten sensitivity.[4] Experts say that this is not a real diagnosis and that there are other factors that may contribute to their symptoms besides a gluten intolerance. Therefore, trying to figure out exactly how many people actually do have a gluten intolerance is difficult.

Whether or not you have been diagnosed with a gluten intolerance, if you have a thyroid problem, it is highly likely that gluten is not good for you, given the fact that 90 percent of thyroid issues are autoimmune in nature. Research backs up the fact that gluten is a very real trigger for autoimmune disease.

How Processing and Modern Eating Patterns Contribute to Disease

Although I do advocate a gluten-free diet when it comes to hypothyroidism, it is also important to understand how processing of wheat and modern eating patterns have contributed to the rise in chronic disease we see today.

The Westernized diet is saturated with foods that are high in processed white flour. If I were to take diet recalls of most people living in affluent countries, they would be filled with foods like sliced bread, bagels, scones, English muffins, pizza, pasta, pastries, and muffins. In fact, when I tell people to try to be gluten-free for a while, it's like I have told them that their favorite pet has died. This lifestyle shows that we have become dependent on fast and easy options instead of taking the time to choose and prepare real, whole foods. In fact, once gluten-containing foods are removed from one's diet, one is forced (in a good way) to start becoming part of the process in terms of acquiring real food that is nutrient dense.

What do I mean by this? I once had a client who really needed to become gluten-free. Her diet was filled with sugar and highly processed white flour. Once I told her to get rid of gluten, she began to eat salads, vegetables, and grass-fed, free-range chicken in the place of her usual sandwich. She switched her afternoon snack of biscuits for fruit and nuts. She ate avocados instead of croutons. All of a sudden, instead of eating nutrition-less processed foods, she began to eat viable, nutrient-dense foods. This is exactly what we need to do in order to support the healing process when thyroid disease is concerned.

To help you understand how processed our diet has become, I believe it is important to understand how the production and processing of wheat has evolved over time. In looking at this, you will begin to have a better appreciation of how our processed diets are destroying our health. Below, I outline the difference between ancient and modern wheat, how wheat is processed to make foods like bread and muffins and what types of additives are put in processed grains. I will also provide recommendations for how to follow a gluten-free lifestyle.

Ancient Wheat versus Modern Wheat

Humans have been eating grains for thousands of years. So, why is there such a huge rise in diet-related chronic diseases today, as compared to thousands or even hundreds of years ago? The answer is that modern grains differ from ancient grains because of the types that are grown and the processing techniques that are used today, and therefore modern grains have sub-optimal nutrient density.

Modern wheat, because of genetic modification and cross-breeding, has been turned into high-yield dwarf wheat (making it cost-effective and profitable). It is lower in zinc, copper, iron, magnesium, and selenium than ancient grains such as einkorn, spelt and kamut.[5,6] It also contains the type of gliadin (part of gluten) protein that is harmful to the human intestinal tract. Studies have shown that modern wheat has more of the harmful kind of gluten than its ancient ancestors.[7] In fact, in people with celiac disease, grains like einkorn had no harmful effect on their disease and were better tolerated than rice (a gluten-free grain).[8]

One study that followed twenty-two healthy participants compared kamut (an older variety of wheat) to modern wheat. Overall, the results showed that the people who ate kamut had lower cholesterol and low-density lipoprotein (LDL) levels, higher potassium and magnesium levels and fewer inflammatory markers than the control group (who ate modern wheat).[9]

Another study tested the microbiome of thirty participants while on a diet containing kamut. Including kamut in the diet resulted in anti-inflammatory effects and a decrease in oxidative activity. Different beneficial bacterial strains were seen on a diet that included kamut as compared to a diet that did not.[10]

There definitely needs to be more large-scale research to ascertain what kinds of effects organic ancient grains have on our health. In the case of hypothyroidism or Hashimoto's, there is simply not enough science to justify eating ancient grains as a way to decrease symptoms or to aid in healing.

What Baking Techniques Are Used Today?

In the past, bread was prepared by soaking, fermenting, sprouting and baking with slow-rise yeast. Sprouting and fermenting foods increases their nutritional content. It increases the amino acid lysine (which is vital for producing collagen), reduces anti-nutrients such as phytic acid and lectins, disables enzyme inhibitors and makes nutrients more accessible.[11,12]

To give an example of how these processes can influence human health, one study showed that celiac patients tolerated sourdough bread better than regular modern bread.[13]

How Bread Is Baked Today

Today, wheat is processed by adding bleach (yes, chlorine!) to make it white, and yeast is used instead of slow-rise yeast to bake breads more quickly.

Traditional bread contains four ingredients: flour, water, yeast, and salt. That's it. However, if you have taken the time to look at the ingredients of most store-bought brands of bread, you will find an entire array of toxic ingredients used to enhance taste and to prolong shelf-life.

It's also important to note that a lot of gluten-free processed products also contain deleterious additives. Therefore, just because something is gluten-free does *not* mean that it will help decrease inflammation.

Here are a few common additives to look out for:

Azocarbonamide.

This toxic ingredient is banned in Europe but still used in the United States. It is used as a bread conditioner (A bread conditioner is a chemical that is used to strengthen the texture of a bread or to improve it in some way). It is also the main ingredient in shoe rubber and yoga mats. When it is heated, it becomes carcinogenic. (This gives a new meaning to the toast we eat for breakfast!) I don't think I need to present research to prove that this ingredient is bad for us. Common sense should prevail here.

Polysorbate 80.

Polysorbate 80 is used as an emulsifier in many foods, including baked goods. Research has shown it to negatively affect the immune system and to cause anaphylactic shock. It also causes infertility. The scary part is, this additive is commonly used in many processed foods.

Xantham gum.

Xanthum gum is another emulsifier and is derived from corn. Corn, as well as wheat and soy, is one of the most genetically modified crops in the world. People have been reported to have negative gastrointestinal reactions to xantham gum as well as migraines and skin itchiness.

Mono- and di-glycerides.

This is another emulsifier that is toxic to our health. It is used to improve bread volume. What most people don't know is that these fats are hydrogenated. As you may have read before, hydrogenated oils that form trans fatty acids are linked to increased risk of heart disease and cancer. So, if you innocently buy a loaf of whole-grain bread and think that it is good for you, you may be getting more than you bargained for. In other words, any bread marketed as healthy because it is whole-grain or whole-wheat can be essentially unhealthy because the bread can contain dangerous trans fatty acids in the form of mono- and di-glycerides.

Soy lecithin.

Soy lecithin is a sludge that is a waste product filled with solvents and pesticides that comes from the processing of soy oil. Soy lecithin is bleached with chlorine to make it a more appealing color. This is of concern, first, because the soy that is used in making the soy oil has most likely been genetically modified, and second, because unfermented soy has been linked to digestive distress, immune system breakdown, premenstrual syndrome (PMS), endometriosis, reproductive problems for men and women, allergies, attention deficit disorder (ADD) and attention deficit hyperactivity disorder (ADHD), higher risk of heart disease and cancer and loss of libido. Wow! And the sad part is that soy lecithin is *everywhere* in processed foods.

A recent study published in 2015 found that emulsifiers found in common processed foods were able to change the microbiota of mice.[14] The mice were fed polysorbate 80 and carboxymethylcellulose. Mice with an impaired immune system developed colitis. Mice with a good immune system showed mild inflammation and developed a metabolic disorder that caused them to eat more and become obese, hypoglycemic and insulin resistant.

Why did I include all of the previous information on additives when the subject is a gluten-free diet? Well, I wanted to point out the dangers of eating a diet primarily of processed foods rather than real, whole foods. Additionally, it's important to realize that a lot of dairy- and gluten-free products contain the additives mentioned above. So, again, I emphasize a gluten-free diet made up of real, whole foods, rather than processed "healthy" foods you buy at the supermarket.

What Foods to Avoid and What to Include on a Gluten-Free Diet

As I mentioned earlier, gluten is responsible for regulating molecules that increase intestinal permeability. In someone suffering from Hashimoto's disease, simply removing gluten can put an autoimmune attack into remission. In my experience with patients with thyroid disease, most need to eliminate gluten-containing foods from their diet in order to heal their gut. Since gluten can also trigger an autoimmune response, I advise clients to make their peace with breaking up with gluten forever.

The reason it is wise to exclude gluten entirely from your diet is that even a trace of gluten can trigger an autoimmune attack that can last for up to six months. This means that gluten eaten in January could still be detectable within the blood until June!

It is important to recognize that tests for detecting gluten intolerance or sensitivity may not be very reliable. In people with Hashimoto's, their immune system may be so taxed that it loses its ability to produce antibodies. Therefore, a test may produce a false negative for gluten sensitivity when in fact, gluten intolerance may be very much the case.[15]

Given all of this, it is prudent to take gluten out of the diet and replace it with foods that are nutrient-dense and that will help to put an autoimmune attack into remission and help the thyroid heal.

Foods to Avoid

Here is a list of foods that you should eliminate from your diet when going gluten-free:

- Anything that contains wheat, rye, or barley
- Bread
- Pasta, orzo
- Crackers
- Bulgar wheat
- Muffins
- Cakes
- Doughnuts
- Biscuits, cookies
- Bagels
- English muffins
- Pancakes, crepes
- Bread crumbs
- Brewer's yeast
- Breading
- Soup bases and bouillons

The previous food mentioned are obvious sources of gluten.

Here is a list of foods that, though less obvious, may also contain gluten:

- Soy sauce (unless it's labelled wheat- or gluten-free)
- Sauces of all types like marinades, gravies, and salad dressings
- French fries or crisps sometimes (they may have flour added to them)
- Spice mixtures (they may use wheat as a filler or anti-caking agent)
- Processed cereals (they may have barley malt in them)
- Ice cream (it may have flour in it)
- Rice or soy milk (they may contain barley)
- Beer (unless it's gluten-free)
- Processed deli meats
- Stuffings
- Barley malt
- Breading
- Brewer's yeast
- Coating mixes
- Croutons
- Malt
- Malt vinegar
- Panko (bread crumbs)
- Soup bases and bouillon

- Syrups

- Thickeners

- Foods sold in bulk (these are often contaminated by scoops used in other bins, and possibly by flour floating around in the air)

- Asian rice paper

- Vitamin E (or any other supplement that can use wheat germ as its source)

I find that the easiest way to be gluten-free is to prepare your own food and to choose real, whole foods instead of processed foods. If you do choose to get pre-packaged foods, read the labels carefully. Look for these words on the label, as these products do contain gluten:

wheat, rye, barley, oats, atta flour, bran, bleached or unbleached flour, barley grass, bread flour, bulgar, cous cous, dinkle (spelt), durham, einkorn, emmer (durham wheat), farina, farro (called emmer wheat except in Italy), food starch, fu (a dried form of gluten), gliadin, gluten, gluten peptides, glutenin, graham, hydrolyzed wheat protein, hydrolyzed wheat gluten, kamut, maida (Indian wheat flour), matza (matso, matsoh), mir (a wheat and rye cross), seitan (gluten), semolina, spelt, starch, triticale, wheat bran, wheat germ, wheat grass, wheat starch.

Cross-Contamination

Gluten is made up of a group of proteins that are not degraded by heat or destroyed by cutting or shaking. This means that if someone brings you a salad with croutons on it, you cannot just pick the croutons off and eat the salad. There will still be gluten particles on the salad, rendering it *not* gluten-free.

Here are a few things to consider in order to avoid cross-contamination in your home:

- If not everyone in your house is gluten-free, make sure to use separate cutting boards and utensils for food preparation. The most obvious household appliance that needs to be segregated is the toaster. Definitely do not use the same toaster for gluten-free breads and regular breads. Gluten can also reside in scrapes in Tupperware, so be sure to use a specific color to denote a gluten-free container.
- Use separate condiments. If a squeeze bottle touches a bun or a pita, it is contaminated and is no longer gluten-free.
- Check your beauty products for gluten. This may sound extreme, but if you use a cream that contains gluten and forget to wash your hands, you could easily contaminate yourself. It's impossible to read the labels of beauty products, as many don't make any sense, so choose beauty

products from a company that specifically makes gluten-free products.

- Use separate sponges for washing up, as again, cross-contamination can occur.

- Don't assume that foods that are naturally gluten-free, such as rice quinoa, corn, or kidney beans, actually *are* gluten free. If a food is not labelled as gluten-free, there may be cross-contamination issues. From harvest to processing, foods can be contaminated with gluten.

Foods to Include

Here are some foods to include on a gluten-free diet:

- Fresh or frozen fruits and vegetables
- Starchy vegetables like sweet potato
- Grass-fed organic meats and poultry
- Grains like quinoa or millet (these are gluten-free, but typically not on an autoimmune protocol)
- Grass-fed organic dairy (unless you are lactose-intolerant or have a casein or whey intolerance)
- Nuts and seeds (unless your leaky gut is severe or you have an intolerance)
- Fish and seafood
- Coconut milk and oil, olive oil

- Free-range, organic eggs (unless you are intolerant or have an allergy)

Remember that the above are only general recommendations, as everyone is different and requires different foods to heal. However, this does give you a point from which to begin. If you are unsure about these foods, please do not hesitate to find a functional medicine practitioner or a nutritionist knowledgeable in gluten-free diets to tailor a meal plan specifically for you.

What Elimination Diets Can Offer

How do you know that gluten is not for you? As mentioned previously, gluten intolerance testing can be inconclusive and expensive. However, an easy and cheap way to see if you are intolerant to a food is to try an elimination diet. What this entails is eliminating foods you suspect you might be intolerant to for two weeks to one month, and then reintroducing them one at a time to see if symptoms reappear.

For example, if you decide to eliminate gluten and dairy from your diet for two weeks, you will first reintroduce gluten. If you experience some symptoms, you know that you have to exclude gluten from your diet. Three days later, you will reintroduce dairy, and again, if symptoms appear, you will know you need to exclude dairy as well. If no symptoms appear, you can continue to include gluten and dairy in your diet. In my experience, however, the most common intolerances are to gluten and dairy. Many people see great improvements in their health and appearance simply by cutting these foods out of their diets.

After being gluten- and dairy-free for a while, reintroducing foods can have different effects on different people. For example, when I tried to eat yogurt from goat's and cow's milk, I immediately became bloated. There will therefore be a lot of trial and error with what you can tolerate as you heal.

Case Study

A seventy-two year-old woman came to me to lose weight but also stated that she had such severe arthritis (another common autoimmune disorder) in her hands, that she could barely move them.

I put her on a strict gluten-free diet and didn't change any of her other eating habits. After only *one week*, she came into my office and said, "Look!" while showing me that she was able to move her hands for the first time in years!

In this case, it was obvious that gluten was causing the inflammation in her body. Needless to say, this lifestyle change helped her to lose weight and to gain energy, things she had not been able to accomplish in a long time.

The Truth About Soy and Other Goitrogens

Soy

It has been well documented for decades that soy inhibits
thyroid function. It does so because the phytoestrogens (plant-
based estrogens that mimic natural estrogens within the human
body) block the production of T3 and T4 by inhibiting thyroid
peroxidase. The specific goitrogens in soy that inhibit thyroid
hormone production are genistein, daidzein and glycitein and
they are not destroyed by cooking.[16]

A 2012 study that followed two newborns with congenital
hypothyroidism showed a marked decrease in thyroid function
when the infants were given soy milk and thyroxine together.
When use of soy milk was stopped, thyroid function
improved.[17]

As there is not sufficient research to assess the dangers of soy
on the thyroid, I typically recommend that clients with
hypothyroidism avoid soy or soy products altogether.

Are Goitrogens Really Bad for Thyroid Function?

Goitrogens are substances that can hinder thyroid function by
interfering with iodine uptake. They are found in cruciferous

vegetables like broccoli, cauliflower, and sweet potatoes. (See complete list below.)

Although the idea that eating goitrogens can cause thyroid problems is quite popular amongst conventional and alternative health care practitioners, the truth is that there is no proof that goitrogens interfere with thyroid function when no iodine deficiency is present. If iodine and selenium are deficient, eating goitrogenic foods can then be a problem. Since iodine and selenium work synergistically, one should rule out an iodine or selenium deficiency before eating goitrogen-containing foods.

In my opinion, if you cut out cruciferous vegetables or other fruits that contain goitrogens, you are missing out on an entire array of antioxidant and anti-cancer properties found in these kinds of foods.

A clinical trial evaluating the safety of isothiocyanates (goitrogenic substances found in cruciferous vegetables) isolated from broccoli sprouts showed that there were no adverse effects (including no effect on thyroid function).[18] There is also research that shows thiocyanates at low concentrations actually stimulate T4 synthesis, supporting the thyroid instead of diminishing its function.[19]

It is also important to note that goitrogens can be deactivated by cooking. Therefore, while you correct for any iodine or selenium deficiencies you can enjoy cruciferous vegetables cooked. Once you are no longer deficient, feel free to enjoy your vegetables raw.

Goitrogen-Containing Foods

Arugula (aka rocket)	Chinese Broccoli	Kale	Rapini (broccoli rabe)
Bok Choy	Collard greens	Kohlrabi	Rutabaga
Broccoli	Daikon	Komatsun and cress	Tatsoi
Broccoflower	Field pepperweed	Maca	Turnip
Brussel Sprouts	Flowering cabbage	Mizuna	Wasabi
Cabbage	Garden cress	Mustard	Watercress
Cauliflower	Horseradish	Radish	Wild broccoli

Adapted from *The Paleo Approach* by Sarah Ballantyne, PhD

Is Being Vegan a Good Idea for Healing Hypothyroidism?

I often have friendly debates with colleagues who believe in a vegan lifestyle. Although there is a lot of research that shows us that, in general, vegans have decreased risk for cancer and heart disease and live longer than their omnivore counterparts, a vegan lifestyle is counter-indicated in attempting to heal a thyroid issue.

In my own experience, when I tried to follow a vegan protocol, my symptoms of fatigue, weakness, dizziness, and lethargy increased. I would always question why other people who followed a vegan diet were able to have so much energy and to even run marathons while I could not, so I began to research the subject.

What I found was that a vegan diet can exacerbate a thyroid disorder. This is so for many different reasons. As we have seen, hypothyroidism can have its root cause in the intestines, in the adrenals, in hormone imbalance or in other areas. In order to alleviate a lot of these issues, many nutrients that are not found in a typical vegan diet are needed.

Vitamin B12

Vitamin B12 or cobalamine is a water-soluble vitamin that is essential in brain and nervous system function and in red blood cell production. It decreases homocysteine, a protein that, when elevated, can be indicative of higher risk of heart disease in the blood.

Very low levels can lead to pernicious anemia and can impair digestion and produce underdeveloped villi in the small intestine.

In What Foods Is Vitamin B12 Abundant?

Vitamin B12 is found primarily in foods like meat, poultry, dairy, eggs and shellfish. Obviously, if you are vegan, you won't eat these foods and you run the risk of being deficient in this very important vitamin. Hypothyroid patients are already at risk for decreased absorption due to having decreased stomach acid. Not eating good sources of B12 simply exacerbates the problem.

How Is Vitamin B12 Absorbed?

In order for vitamin B12 to be absorbed, there must be enough intrinsic factor present within the stomach. Intrinsic factor is responsible for removing vitamin B12 from its protein source in order for it to be absorbed further down in the large intestine. In order for there to be enough intrinsic factor, there must be enough stomach acid available. I often recommend a stomach acid supplement along with digestive enzymes in order to enhance vitamin B12 absorption. (Read more about vitamin

B12 in chapter 5).

Iron/Ferritin

One of the most important functions of iron is for the transport of oxygen to all the cells in the body. This is why one feels fatigue when iron levels are low; not enough oxygen is readily available for the cells to function.

Typically, low iron stores are diagnosed by your doctor via hemoglobin, hematocrit and iron concentration. However, it is important to know ferritin (the storage form of iron) levels in order to determine proper levels of iron.

Knowing how important iron is, the issue of absorption becomes especially important. Although there are vegan foods, like spinach, lentils and swiss chard, that are higher in iron, and a vegan diet typically is a good source of vitamin C, which increases the absorption of these iron sources, the absorption of iron with a vegan diet when one has hypothyroidism is again hindered.

Why is this? Vegans believe in eating most of their foods raw . Raw vegetables, grains, legumes, and nuts are higher in a substance called phytic acid which can cause more irritation on an inflamed intestine and also decreases the absorption of vitamins and minerals like iron. If the intestine is impaired, it cannot extract iron from vegan food sources.

As we have seen, hypothyroidism patients typically need to heal a leaky gut in order to resolve any hypothyroid symptoms. In order to heal the gut, most vegetables, and sometimes fruits as well, need to be cooked in order to break down phytic acid content and decrease extra irritation to the intestinal lining. A raw vegan lifestyle would not be conducive to this.

Iron from organic sources of foods like beef and chicken are much more readily absorbed than from vegan sources. Again, enough stomach acid needs to be present in order for successful iron absorption.

Carbohydrate- versus Protein-Rich Diet

A vegan diet is predominantly made up of carbohydrate-rich foods and deficient in the high amount of amino acids that are needed to fix and repair vital organs (intestines, adrenal glands, thyroid, etc.) This could be detrimental to healing the thyroid gland for two reasons:

First, as mentioned previously, if there are blood sugar issues that need to be addressed, a high-carbohydrate diet is not indicated. Although the high fiber content found in a vegan diet can decrease the rate of absorption of glucose, more protein is still needed to balance blood sugar issues.

Second, more available amino acids are needed to support the healing of vital organs such as the intestine and the thyroid gland as well as to support detoxification processes. A vegan diet cannot provide the therapeutic levels of amino acids needed.

Let's take the amino acid lysine, for example. Lysine is needed to promote collagen synthesis. For a healthy person, 12 milligrams of collagen per kilogram of body weight is recommended, which means that for the average 70 kg person, 840 mg per day is needed.

One hundred grams of bone broth has 4.4 grams (or 4,400mg) of lysine. In order to get that amount with kale, you would need to eat thirty cups of it. You begin to see why a vegan diet would be limiting when trying to heal.

An Omnivore Diet May Enhance the Microbiome and Decrease Inflammation

Another recent finding in research is that people who are not vegetarian have a higher number of good bacteria in their gut. A 2015 study published in Scientific Reports found that mice fed different diets (vegetarian, red meat or white meat) had marked differences in the biodiversity of their microbiome.21 This suggested that people who eat meat-sourced protein have a more balanced composition of gut bacteria. This contributes to less inflammation in the body.

As with all chronic diseases, decreasing inflammation is very important when we want to promote thyroid function. It seems that, once again, being a vegetarian may not help the thyroid to work optimally.

Non-food Considerations for Thyroid Health

Thyroid health is not just about the food you eat. It is also about the products, chemicals and water that you choose to use on your skin and hair. It is proposed that women have a higher occurrence of thyroid issues because of the many things they apply on a daily basis, such as creams, make-up, shampoos and perfumes. In my experience, I always noticed that my skin would break out in acne with anything that I would apply on my face. It took me a while to realize how sensitive I was to all of the chemicals that are found in common cosmetics.

Common household cleaning products can also have serious affects on thyroid health. Below, I outline a few of the products you should be wary of and where to look to find more natural products.

Beauty Is From within: Throw Out Those Cosmetics and Creams!

It is often quite a shock to find out that our favourite creams and shampoos are laden with toxic chemicals that could impair thyroid function (or even worse, cause cancer). At this point, however, it should come as no surprise that all the chemicals you see on the back of popular cosmetics have side effects.

Keep in mind that there are many chemicals that you should be wary of, but I chose a few that relate to the thyroid specifically.

Octinoxate

Octinoxate is a chemical that is an ultraviolet filter and is absorbed easily through the skin. Since this is so, this toxin can be found in the blood and urine of humans after its use. It is a hormone disruptor as it mimics estrogen and disrupts the proper functioning of the thyroid. Octinoxate is typically found in hair color products, shampoos, sunscreen, lipstick, nail polish and skin creams. (That's quite a list!)

Resorcinol

In high doses, resorcinol can be toxic and can lead to respiratory issues. It is an endocrine disruptor and specifically has a bad effect on thyroid function. Resorcinol is commonly found in hair dyes, shampoos, hair lotions and peels and products used to treat acne, eczema and other dermatological issues. (Of course, healing the gut could help to reverse these skin issues without these products.)

Parabens

Parabens are used in many cosmetics and food products to decrease the growth of microbes. They can be absorbed through the skin, blood and digestive system and are endocrine disruptors. They are commonly found in shampoos, conditioners, lotions and facial and shower cleansers and scrubs.

The above is by no means an extensive list of chemicals. I shared it so that you can appreciate how something seemingly harmless, can have a major impact on health. For an in-depth look at chemicals commonly found in everyday cosmetics as well as a list of safe cosmetics for everyday use, check out www.safecosmetics.org. Also, take a look at the environmental working group's web page as they rate over eight thousand products in terms of consumer health safety (www.ewr.org.)

Common Household Products to Avoid

Plastic

Plastic is hazardous to thyroid function. A chemical called antimony leaches from plastic bottles and is often found in drinks or water that are contained in them over a long period of time. Phthalates found in plastic bottles are known to affect thyroid function.

Flame Retardants

These chemicals are found in the screens of televisions and computers and can disrupt the proper functioning of the thyroid.

Non stick Surfaces

The chemical that is found in a non-stick frying pan or used in certain food packages can definitely negatively affect your thyroid. Only moderate exposure is enough to trigger thyroid dysfunction.

Products Containing Triclosan

As will be mentioned in chapter five, triclosan interferes with the hormones produced by the thyroid as well as with estrogen and testosterone levels. It is found in products like dishwashing liquid, hand soap and toothpaste.

Chlorine

Chlorine can not only be found in the bleach you use to clean toilets but it is also present in drinking water as well the water you use to take a shower. Chlorine that contains PCBs (polychlorinated biphenyls) is yet another powerful endocrine disruptor and is toxic to thyroid cells. PCBs increase TSH, thyroid antibodies and thyroid size.

In order to avoid chlorine in the home, use a water filter for your drinking water as well as for the shower head, as chlorine can be absorbed through the skin. Obviously, inhaling fumes from chlorine use as a cleaning agent should be avoided.

Is Excessive Exercise Making You Sick?

The scientific literature shows an obvious connection between physical activity and good health. It helps to prevent diseases like type 2 diabetes, heart disease and cancer and helps to regulate various hormones within the body. Being sedentary increases one's chance of disease development and mortality.

When it comes to the thyroid and autoimmune disease, however, exercise needs to be looked at this way: too little or too much can cause disease. Excessive aerobic or interval training can increase cortisol levels and result in adrenal insufficiency, a leaky gut and susceptibility to an autoimmune condition.

When I was really pushing myself to run 10 kilometers or to do interval training every day, I felt really sick, run-down and exhausted. I would not get the runner's high or the adrenaline rush that other athletes or gym-goers spoke of. I found out that finding the right type of exercise is essential to good health.

Finding the right way to exercise to balance the immune system is dependent on several factors:

- Type of activity (aerobic or weight training)
- Duration and intensity of activity
- Time of day
- Whether or not you exercise on an empty stomach
- How long it has been since you previously exercised
- Whether or not you exercise regularly

Acute exercise (which means doing more than you are used to in terms of duration and/or intensity or doing exercise once in a while) stimulates inflammation. This obviously can exacerbate an autoimmune condition. If you exercise regularly, however, some studies have shown an anti-inflammatory effect (but other studies have shown an inflammatory effect once again).

If you have a thyroid condition, it is very important to implement low-to moderate- intensity physical activity as a lifestyle. It is also imperative to consider that exercising for an autoimmune condition should not be about looking like a model. It should be about health. Therefore, if you choose a form of exercise that just makes you feel worse (like me with running), you should abstain from it and find something that boosts your energy and makes you feel better overall. For me, I found that balance with some light weight training, walking and yoga or pilates.

I am not a fitness expert, and I cannot give you a more in-depth look at what types of physical activities can benefit your thyroid. I wanted to mention exercise, however, because it is a crucial part of healing. Therefore, use this information to talk with a trained holistic exercise physiologist to find out what exercise works best for you.

CHAPTER 5

DIETS AND FOODS TO CONSIDER FOR HYPOTHYROIDISM

Can a detox Help to Boost Thyroid Function?

Detox has become a very popular topic of discussion within mainstream nutrition. Here, it becomes important to understand that there are always opportunistic people who follow the trends in order to offer quick fixes and non-scientific solutions in order to make some money. The detox trend is no exception. Therefore, in this chapter I will outline what a detox is and the research on some foods and supplements that help the body with its own detoxification process. This way you can make more educated decisions about what detox options you decide to pursue.

Having said this, however, detox can serve as a great means to rid the body of toxins that exist (even for a lifetime) in the body. Many toxins found in drugs, pesticides, insecticides, synthetic hormones and the like, can build up in fatty tissue and cause problems as serious as cancer. Toxins obviously can cause problems for the thyroid as well.

Toxins that Suppress Thyroid Function

In this book, I have already outlined how nutrition can help boost thyroid function. However, I would remiss not to mention the environmental toxins that a lot of us are exposed to daily that can have a negative impact on thyroid health. A thyroid problem could very well be caused by a number of these different toxins.

I have already mentioned a few toxins that reduce thyroid function in chapter three, however, I have also included the following, which has been adapted from Dr. William Cole, a functional medicine practitioner who specializes in thyroid issues.

Perchlorates

This toxin leaks into our food and water supply and is a byproduct of things like jet fuel and fireworks. It prevents the production of thyroid hormone.

Polychlorinated Biphenyls (PCBs)

Polychlorinated biphenyls are banned chemicals (still present in the environment) that can block thyroid function by making your body resistant to thyroid hormone. They can also interfere with liver enzymes which can further inhibit the production of active thyroid hormone.

Dioxins

These toxins have also been noted to be endocrine disrupters and affect thyroid function.

Soy

Soy contains phytoestrogens, which are known to block the enzyme thyroid peroxidase. It also blocks the conversion of iodine to thyroid hormone and therefore the conversion of T4 to T3.

Pesticides

Pesticides in general decrease thyroid function. Certain weed killers and anti-fungals have been shown to decrease thyroid function and cause weight loss resistance.

Flame Retardants

These disturb thyroid function and can be found in television and computer screens.

Plastics

Things like bisphenoal-A (BPA) found in plastics and dental sealants have been found to cause thyroid hormone resistance by decreasing thyroid receptor site sensitivity.

Perfluorooctanoic Acid (PFOA)

Perfluorooctanoic acid, a substance found in things like Teflon, has been shown to negatively affect thyroid function.

Halogens

Fluoride and chloride are known to suppress the conversion of T4 to T3 (the active form of thyroid hormone). The amount of fluoride needed to decrease thyroid function is low, 2 to 5 milligrams per day. Fluoride and chloride can also occupy your iodine receptors, making it impossible for you to properly use iodine.

Heavy Metals

Mercury, lead, and aluminium can trigger an autoimmune attack, such as with Hashimoto's thyroiditis. According to Dr. William Cole, people can have "a chronic heavy metal toxicity which can only be accurately shown with a urine test using a chelating agent. The chelator will pull the metals from your cells where it has leached, so it can actually be measured on the test."

Antibacterial products

The antibacterial chemical Triclosan that is commonly used in things like soaps is an endocrine disruptor and can have an effect on thyroid hormones.

How Detox Can Help

There are many detox regimens that include the use of specific herbs, plants, and foods in general that support the natural detoxification pathways of the body. A detox program should always be done under the supervision of a health professional trained in this area.

The Two Stages of the Body's Natural Detoxification Process

The large intestine, the liver, the skin, and the lungs are all designed to get rid of toxins. The main detoxification processes of the body, however, take place in the liver and can be categorized in two phases: phase 1 and phase 2 detoxification.

In very simplistic terms, phase 1 detoxification breaks down toxins and phase 2 detoxification removes the toxins from the body.

In phase 1 detoxification, the liver turns toxic chemicals into less toxic chemicals. However, if there are not sufficient amounts of antioxidants available (like vitamin C, vitamin E, or carotenoids), the free radicals formed by this process build up within the liver cells and can actually destroy them.

In phase 2 detoxification, antioxidants like glutathione or amino acids like glycine, attach to the toxins, make them water-soluble, and are excreted in fluids like urine from the body.

As one can see, the detoxification process needs proper nutrition in order to effectively work. If you have deficiencies or your immune system is suppressed in any way, the detoxification process is hindered. So, effectively, this is what a proper detox will do. It will provide the nutrition necessary to increase the body's ability to get rid of toxins. It's as simple as that.

What Kind of Detox Should You Follow?

It is obviously beyond the scope of this book to recommend specific detoxes to each individual. Detox recommendations vary greatly according to a person's health status. However, there are some things to watch out for if you have hypothyroidism.

What to Consider in a Detox When You Have Hypothyroidism

As over 90 percent of hypothyroidism cases are related to an autoimmune condition, it is important to understand which common detox foods and practices may exacerbate a thyroid disorder.

Here are a few general recommendations to help you to get on the right track as it applies to thyroid health:

1. *Heal your gut.* No amount of detox will be beneficial if your digestive tract has dysbiosis or is not functioning optimally. (Please refer back to chapter 2).

2. *Start slowly.* If you have been unwell for a while, I would suggest starting with an elimination diet first to decrease inflammation. For example, try eliminating wheat, dairy and all processed foods from your diet. This will help your body to slowly transition to better health without overwhelming it with a powerful detox plan.

3. *Add back real foods.* Add foods into your daily regimen that are nutrient dense and that will help support the optimal functioning of the thyroid. These include fruits, vegetables, grass-fed organic meats and poultry, wild-caught fish, nuts and seeds.

4. *Use supplements.* Start using detox foods or supplements one month after starting an elimination diet.

5. *Avoid common detox foods such as spirulina or chlorella.* Although they are known for binding toxins, they are also immune stimulators and may exacerbate an autoimmune condition.

6. *Avoid Fasting.* Fasting (a common tactic used in many detoxification schemes) for long periods of time may be counter indicated for hypothyroid patients as many have

157

issues with adrenal insufficiency or blood glucose imbalance. Fasting can exacerbate a hypothyroid problem. Therefore, try to follow a detox program that focuses on enhancing your own detoxification capabilities with natural foods rather than on going without food for long periods of time.

The reason it is important to detox slowly, especially when you have several health issues going on, is that a strong detox can have side effects such as weakness, tiredness, nausea, headaches, general aches and pains and dizziness. In order to avoid strong versions of all of these symptoms, taking it slow is key to a proper detox regimen.

Supplements that Help the Liver to Detox:

The following are herbs, foods, vitamins, minerals and other supplements that help the body's natural detoxification processes (foods that can exacerbate an autoimmune condition are also discussed).

Milk Thistle **(Silybum marianum)**

Milk thistle has been known for its antioxidant and anti-inflammatory effects on the liver. It stimulates the growth and regeneration of injured liver cells. Milk thistle supports phase 1 detoxification and prevents the depletion of hepatic glutathione, which is important for phase 2 detoxification.

Alpha-linoleic Acid (ALA)

As will be mentioned later in this chapter, ALA or alpha-linoleic acid is a form of omega-3 fatty acid that is found in foods like flaxseed and hemp oils. It is the precursor to the powerful liver antioxidant glutathione. If you are ALA deficient, chances are you are not producing enough glutathione which is used in phase 2 detoxification. It should be noted, however, that foods such as flaxseed or hemp seed may exacerbate the immune system and should be avoided in some people.

Glutathione and Superoxide Dismutase (SOD)

According to Dr. Kharrazian, author of the book, *Why Do I Still Have Thyroid Symptoms?*, these are "important substrates for hepatic detoxification. Glutathione is important for phase 2 conjugation, and both SOD and glutathione are important for phase 1 oxidation/reduction reactions. When hepatic reserves of glutathione become depleted, detoxification potentials become hindered and the body becomes more susceptible to exogenous and endogenous toxins. Studies have shown that glutathione depletion contributes and is linked to liver disease, cirrhosis, hepatitis, fatty liver, and alcohol-damaged liver."

"The status of glutathione is considered the single most accurate indicator of the health of the cell. Antioxidant levels become depleted in inflammatory and degenerative conditions and their depletions creates a vicious cycle of further oxidative stress and degeneration."

Glutathione and SOD are also very important for the proper functioning of the immune system. Therefore, considering them not only for detox purposes, but for autoimmune disease like Hashimoto's is a very good idea.

Dr. Kharrazian recommends that these two antioxidants be used in a cream and applied to the bottom of the feet for optimal absorption.

Curcumin

Curcumin is a naturally occurring substance in turmeric. It has been well documented for its anti-carcinogenic effects on the body. It also serves a purpose in both detoxification phases.

Curcumin has been found to inhibit phase 1 detoxification and to stimulate phase 2 detoxification. In other words, in the case of carcinogens, it can deactivate carcinogens while increasing the detoxification of those that are activated. In this way, curcumin can help decrease the cancer-causing effects of toxins like tobacco.

Amino acids

Along with alpha-linolenic acid, cysteine and glycine are precursors to glutathione formation in phase 2 detoxification. Studies have shown that supplementing with cysteine and glycine fully restores glutathione synthesis (if depleted) and therefore decreases oxidative stress in the body.[5] If there is not enough glycine present, the liver cannot carry out its normal detoxification process.

Environmental toxins, food preservatives, and bacteria all need glycine to be eliminated from the body. If a person is overloaded with these toxins, he or she should definitely consider a glycine supplement in order to more effectively detox these poisons from his or her body. Don't forget that glycine is the amino acid that is predominantly present in organic bone broth.

For efficient phase two detoxification, the liver cells require sulphur-containing amino acids such as taurine and cysteine. The nutrients glycine, glutamine, choline and inositol are also required for efficient phase two detoxification.

Eggs, cruciferous vegetables (broccoli, cabbage, Brussels sprouts and cauliflower), raw garlic, onions, leeks and shallots are all good sources of natural sulphur compounds to enhance phase two detoxification. Thus, these foods can be considered to have a cleansing action. Remember that foods such as eggs and onions may not be good for everyone with an autoimmune condition.

Bone broth

Recognize this specific food? If you were paying attention in the chapter about healing your gut, this is where it appeared before. Besides being able to form collagen to repair the lining of the intestines, bone broth also helps the liver detoxification processes. This is so because it is rich in a highly absorbable form of the amino acid glycine, which helps with both phase 1 and phase 2 of the detoxification process.

The Importance of Organic

Many experts argue that the food we eat today is starved of essential nutrients. Soils are depleted of minerals like magnesium and selenium and conventional livestock is polluted with antibiotics, hormones and genetically-modified feed. If you are really looking to cleanse your body, it would be in your best interest to invest in organically grown and raised food.

Conventional versus Organic

There are two main concerns when addressing organic versus conventionally grown produce. First, there is some preliminary research that suggests that certain pesticides and insecticides used in conventional farming disrupt the immune system by either suppressing its function or stimulating it in the wrong way. Although further research needs to be done to prove this, it seems wise to decrease the exposure to these chemicals as much as possible.

The other consideration is the soil in which conventional fruits and vegetables are grown. There has been as much as 75 percent decrease in vitamins and minerals in the soil as compared to fifty years ago. This is important, as a lot of these nutrients, including magnesium, zinc, selenium, B-vitamins and vitamin E, are vital for the proper functioning of the thyroid.

In order to make sure that you are getting the best produce possible, form relationships with local farmers who make it a point to tell you about their farming conditions and what soil is used.

If a tight budget is a concern, the Environmental Working Group publishes a list of fruits and vegetables every year, known as the Dirty Dozen, that have the highest pesticide and insecticide content. They also publish a list called the Clean Fifteen which are a list of fruits and vegetables that contain the least pesticide and insecticide.

You can buy conventionally grown fruits and vegetables from the clean fifteen and wash them properly by soaking then in water and vinegar for fifteen minutes. Peeling fruits also decreases their pesticide content.

Only organically grown fruits and vegetables from the dirty dozen should be purchased, in order to avoid extra exposure to toxins.

Below are the Dirty Dozen and Clean Fifteen for 2017:

Dirty Dozen	Clean Fifteen
• Strawberries • Spinach • Nectarines • Apples • Peaches • Pears • Cherries • Grapes • Celery • Tomatoes • Sweet bell peppers • Potatoes	• Sweet corn • Avocados • Pineapples • Cabbage • Onions • Sweet peas (frozen) • Papayas • Asparagus • Mangos • Eggplant • Honeydew melon • Kiwi • Canteloupe • Cauliflower • Grapefruit

What's Wrong with GMO?

GMO is an acronym that stands for genetically-modified organisms. Crops are genetically modified in order to help them withstand certain environmental conditions so that more yield is produced. The problem with this is that genetically-modified foods contain more of the anti nutrients like digestive-enzyme inhibitors that exacerbate autoimmune conditions. Once again, shopping organic as much as possible will help to limit GMO exposure.

Clean Water

There have been horror stories of what can be found in tap water and bottled water alike. According to the Environmental Protection Agency (EPA), the lead found in drinking water contributes to nearly half a million cases of learning disorders among children per year in the United States. Other dangerous substances such as poisons and used medications have also been reported to exist in drinking water.

Bottled water may not be any better, as the source of bottle water is sometimes not as pure as the company that bottles the water makes it out to be. Even more important, phthalates, which are chemicals that seep out of the plastic and into the water, are deleterious to the thyroid and our health in general.

The point of mentioning the above is to point out that the type of water you choose to drink will definitely affect the outcome of a cleansing program. You need to drink plentiful amounts of water to wash out toxins from the body. If the water you drink is a source of those toxins, you may be detoxifying your body without any results.

Sleep

Sleeping is the time when the body boosts the immune system and does maintenance work on itself. If you do not sleep properly, wake up many times during the night, go to bed late or do not get enough hours of quality sleep, your body does not get the chance to properly cleanse itself. In fact, since a lack of sleep is a major stressor of the body, this increases toxic build-up and is counter-indicated when attempting a detox plan.

Considerations for Detox and Your Thyroid:

A lot of detox programs promote the use of supplements or herbs that can affect the thyroid negatively. For example, spirulina and chlorella have been shown to bind toxins and allow them to be removed by the body. However, if you have an autoimmune disorder like Hashimoto's, these algae can stimulate the immune system and cause it to go awry in sensitive individuals. Also, if too much iodine is of concern in the diet, these foods should be avoided.

My recommendation for eating clean in order to boost thyroid function is to "break-up" with foods that cause excess inflammation and therefore sluggishness within the body, the most obvious culprits being most grains and dairy products. Then make it a point to eat a nutrient-dense diet from a variety of real, whole foods. Work with a nutritionist or doctor to add supplements that will support the liver to gently detoxify the body. Do not use detox regimens with many mystery pills without the supervision and the consultation of a health care professional.

The Right Fats to Eat for your Thyroid

The Saturated Fat Myth Debunked

For a long time, old science has led us to believe that saturated fats are bad for us and that polyunsaturated fats are good and heart healthy. People *still* believe that saturated fats cause high cholesterol levels and ultimately heart disease. The truth is that saturated fats are vital for the proper functioning of our cells and organs and can even help us to lose weight!

In 2010, a meta-analysis of prospective epidemiologic studies published in the *American Journal of Clinical Nutrition* showed that there is no significant evidence for concluding that dietary saturated fat is associated with an increased risk of coronary heart disease or cardiovascular disease.[9] In layman's terms, there is no proof that eating saturated fats increases your risk for heart disease.

Major government and food industry agencies have added to the wrongful demonization of saturated fats both amongst consumers and researchers. Dr. Mary Enig, a pioneer researcher in fats, oils, and lipids research, has stated that "ignoring the levels of trans fatty acids in foods has prevented us from having accurate data on fat composition of our diets."[10] In other words, many studies that demonized saturated fat did not take the amount of trans fatty acids also present in the food supply into account in their research. If they had, I'm guessing that their research results would paint a very different picture.

I will not go into why the food industry as well as government- and pharmaceutical-funded studies led us to believe that saturated fats are bad for us. That could be another book in and of itself. Instead, I would like to focus on the research that proves that saturated fat is, in fact, a necessary part of a healthy diet, and why most polyunsaturated fats are not.

What Are Saturated Fats?

From a biochemical point of view, saturated fats are simply fats that are filled with hydrogen atoms and have no double bonds. What this means in plain English is that the biochemical structure of saturated fat allows it to be a solid at room temperature. It can be found in foods like red meat, chicken, dairy products, as well as some tropical plants like coconuts and palm.

What Role Do Saturated Fats Play in Our Bodies?

Once you see the many important functions saturated fats have in the body, you will be better able to grasp why they are not bad for us and why they should be included in the diet. Here are a few of the important functions of saturated fats:

- Saturated fats present in the diet help to lower lipoprotein (a), a marker that when raised in the blood increases one's risk for heart disease.
- Saturated fats (the medium-chain fatty acids) promote fat loss, especially in the abdominal area.
- Saturated fat is required for calcium to be effectively absorbed into bones.
- Saturated fat protects the liver from medicines and alcohol.
- The lungs contain palmitic acid, a saturated fatty acid that helps prevent asthma.
- Saturated fats found in butter and coconut oil (myristic and lauric acids) play a key role in our immune system. Loss of saturated fat in the fighter cells of our immune

system decrease the body's natural ability to fight bacterial and viral infections. Myristic acid also fights off tumors.

- The brain is mostly made of saturated fats and cholesterol. Without enough saturated fat in the diet, your brain will not perform optimally.

- Saturated fats are needed for the proper utilization of essential fatty acids. Elongated omega-3 fatty acids are better retained in the tissues when the diet is rich in saturated fats.

- Saturated 18-carbon stearic acid and 16-carbon palmitic acid are the preferred foods for the heart, which is why the fat around the heart muscle is highly saturated. The heart draws on this reserve of fat in times of stress.

- Short- and medium-chain saturated fatty acids have important antimicrobial properties. They protect us against harmful microorganisms in the digestive tract.

- The scientific evidence, honestly evaluated, does not support the assertion that "artery- clogging" saturated fats cause heart disease. Actually, evaluation of the fat in artery clogs reveals that only about 26 percent is saturated. The rest is unsaturated, of which more than half is polyunsaturated.

- Vitamins A, D, and K2 primarily found in saturated fat-rich animal products such as eggs, butter, and organ meat, are absent from most plant foods. These are essential for heart health, bone strength and immune function.

- Saturated fats are signaling molecules for hormone production.[11,12,13,14]

With all the functions that saturated fats have in the body, one begins to really question why they have been criticized as an unhealthy part of the diet. If we take a look at American history, one hundred years ago people ate full-fat dairy products, including butter, and they ate grass-fed, free-range eggs. During this time, there was no obesity epidemic and very little heart disease. As soon as the decision was made to make the general public believe that saturated fats were bad and that highly-processed and cheap polyunsaturated fats like soy, corn, sunflower and safflower oils were good, obesity and heart disease sharply increased.

Here is more research that confirms the benefits of saturated fats in the diet:

After reviewing well-designed studies, Harvard researchers in 2010 found that saturated fatty acids improved the total cholesterol to high-density lipoprotein (HDL) ratio in comparison to carbohydrate replacement foods.[15] In other words, eating saturated fats decreases your risk of developing heart disease.

The Sydney Diet Heart Study, conducted from 1966 to 1973, followed 458 middle-aged men who had had a recent coronary event (i.e..,high-risk individuals, to see the effect of a high-saturated-fat diet versus a high-polyunsaturated-fat diet. The researchers found that those consuming the unsaturated fats experienced greater overall mortality than those consuming the saturated fats. The authors suggest that the mechanism of action was enhanced oxidation of the oils, the deleterious effect being most pronounced in smokers and heavy consumers of alcohol, whose oxidative stress is already increased.[16]

The Framingham Study that has followed thousands of people and their offspring in Massachusetts since 1948 has had a very important finding:

The more saturated fat one eats, the more cholesterol one eats, the more calories one eats, the lower one's serum cholesterol.

Saturated Fats Regulate Hormonal Function

As previously mentioned, saturated fats are involved with hormonal signalling throughout the body. Although the body can produce saturated fats, if you do not get enough from your diet, hormonal pathways can suffer and not function properly.

Myristic, stearic, palmitic, lauric and caprylic acids are all saturated fatty acids that are vital to optimal cell functioning.

All of these fatty acids play an important role in signalling important messages from the outside of the cell to the inside of the cell. For example, these saturated fatty acids can be used by our cells to signal the production and use of hormones such as progesterone, adrenaline, and cortisol. As mentioned in previous chapters, all of these hormones are vital for proper functioning of the sexual organs, the adrenal glands, and the thyroid. They are interrelated and like a cascade, if one link is missing, the cascade becomes faulty and the normal flow is interrupted. Therefore, it is very important to get the right amount of saturated fats from our diet for optimal functioning of our hormones.

In order for the body to function properly, we need to get 25 percent of calories from saturated fat. From where can we get this saturated fat in the diet? The following list explains the benefits of each source of saturated fat.

Foods That Boost Thyroid Function

Raw Cacao

Raw cacao contains 35 percent stearic acid and 25 percent palmitic acid. Both have been shown by research to lower cholesterol levels. There is also preliminary research that cacao can have a positive effect on blood flow and has a very high antioxidant capacity that can promote longevity and well-being.[20,21] Although cacao may be counter-indicated in an autoimmune protocol, I would add some back with caution once symptoms improve.

Grass-Fed Butter

Butter contains large amounts of the saturated fatty acid butyrate. Studies have shown that butyrate has a large anti-inflammatory effect on the body.[22] Therefore, grass-fed butter has the capability of decreasing your risk for diseases associated with increased inflammation such as heart disease and diabetes.

Butyrate is also responsible for increasing the number of thyroid hormone receptors. This allows your cells to use more thyroid hormone.[23]

Grass-fed butter is a very good source of vitamin K2. There is evidence that good amounts of vitamin K2 dramatically decrease one's chances of developing diseases such as osteoporosis and heart disease.

Although dairy products are usually avoided on an autoimmune protocol, from my experience, I find that butter is the only dairy product that is tolerated by my patients.

Grass-Fed Beef

Beef that is either grain or grass fed contains three saturated fatty acids: stearic, myristic and palmitic. Grass-fed beef, however, is higher in stearic acid, which has the ability to lower cholesterol levels.

As far as polyunsaturated fats are concerned, grass-fed beef has a better omega-6 to omega-3 ratio. Conventionally raised beef has a ratio of nearly 8:1 whereas grass-fed beef's ratio is about 1.5:1. In order for omega-6 and omega-3 fatty acids to co-exist in a healthy diet, the ratio should be as close to 1:1 as possible. (More on the omega-6 to omega-3 ratio later.)

Grass-fed beef is also two to three times higher in a polyunsaturated fat called conjugated linoleic acid which has been shown by research to have great antioxidant capacity.

Grass-fed beef contains more of the antioxidants vitamin E, glutathione, superoxide dismutase (SOD), and catalase than grain-fed beef. These antioxidants play an important role in protecting our cells from oxidation, especially fats in the cell membrane such as omega-3 and omega-6. Also, grass-fed beef has more carotenoids, which makes the fat look more yellow. Therefore, a great way to tell if your meat is more nutrient dense is simply by looking at the color.[30,31,32]

Egg Yolks

Besides being a powerhouse of nutrition rich in B-vitamins, vitamin A, selenium and folate (to name a few), grass-fed eggs are higher in omega-3 fatty acids. As with beef, the feed of the chicken affects whether or not the eggs will have sufficient omega-3 content. Therefore, it is always important to choose free-range eggs.

Many people with autoimmune disease cannot tolerate the whites of eggs. I usually recommend only the yolks to be used when one has autoimmune thyroid disease.

Coconut Oil

Coconut oil is 90 percent saturated fat and contains both lauric and caprylic fatty acids. Both of these fatty acids have antifungal, antibacterial and antiviral properties that allow them to increase the power of the immune system. This is also good news for creating a better environment in our gastrointestinal tracts, as coconut oil can kill off dangerous bacteria like *Staphylococcus aureus* and fungi like *Candida albicans*. Coconut oil also contains medium-chain triglycerides which help to decrease abdominal fat and provide a good source of energy as they go straight to the liver to be metabolized.[33,34,35,36]

Olive Oil

Extra virgin olive oil has 73 percent monounsaturated fats in the form of oleic acid. It has a high phenolic content that provides most of its health benefits as a potent antioxidant. Oleic acid itself can reduce inflammation. The phenolic compounds that act as antioxidants, oleocanthal and oleuropein, have been found to have similar anti-inflammatory effects with the drug ibuprofen.[37,38,39,40,41,42]

Flaxseed Oil

Flaxseed oil is concentrated with omega-3 fatty acids in the form of alpha-linolenic acid or ALA. ALA is a super antioxidant that can help to form other important antioxidants in the body, like vitamins C and E and glutathione. This means that when these antioxidants run out, if there is ALA present, they can be reformed. ALA is also the only free fatty acid that is known to be able to get into your brain and therefore it has been used by some doctors to treat the after effects of a stroke.

There is also research that suggests that ALA can be used to treat autoimmune disease. This is great news for people with Hashimoto's disease, as ALA can help boost the immune system to reduce the severity of an attack on the thyroid.

Flaxseed oil also contains lignans, which block estrogen

receptors in the body and therefore reduce the estrogenic stimulation of the body. Therefore, they may be useful in reducing the size of tumors in breast and prostate cancer. This also helps the thyroid as estrogen works against the proper functioning of the thyroid (as discussed earlier).

Lignans also help to maintain a stable blood glucose level, help to reduce cholesterol levels, and can help to alleviate constipation (therefore helping to heal the gut, something that is necessary for proper thyroid function).

Although flaxseed may be a good source of ALA, it is not typically used by those on an autoimmune protocol because it is not easily absorbed by the body and feeds bacteria known to exacerbate gut inflammation.

Please note that ALA can also be found in hemp and chia seeds.

What Polyunsaturated Fats *Should* There Be in the Diet?

Why Are Polyunsaturated Fats Dangerous?

In the following text, Dr. Enig explains why highly processed polyunsaturated oils like canola, sunflower, safflower, soy and the like are deleterious to our health:

"Excess consumption of polyunsaturated oils has been shown to contribute to a large number of disease conditions including increased cancer and heart disease; immune system dysfunction; damage to the liver, reproductive organs and lungs; digestive disorders; depressed learning ability; impaired growth; and weight gain.

"Rancid oils from polyunsaturated fats create free radicals that attack cell membranes and red blood cells and cause damage in DNA/RNA strands, thus triggering mutations in tissue, blood vessels and skin. Free radical damage to the skin causes wrinkles and premature aging; free radical damage to the tissues and organs sets the stage for tumors; free radical damage in the blood vessels initiates the buildup of plaque. New evidence links exposure to free radicals with premature aging, with autoimmune diseases such as arthritis and with Parkinson's disease, Lou Gehrig's disease, Alzheimer's and cataracts."

Most of these polyunsaturated fats are found in the highly processed Westernized diet we are used to today. There is no wonder that there is such an increase in disease related to obesity and endocrine dysfunction as there is in this day and age.

What about Omega-3 Fatty Acids? Those Are Supposed to Be Good Polyunsaturated Fats, Right?

Yes, they are good forms of polyunsaturated fats. They are important for cell oxidation and for maintaining proper prostaglandin balance (allowing them to have an anti-inflammatory effect). However, with the increase of highly processed oils such as sunflower, safflower, soy, and canola, there is also a huge increase in the amount of omega-6 fatty acids and a decrease in omega-3 fatty acids in the diet. Omega-6 fatty acids interfere with the production of important prostaglandins. "This disruption can result in increased tendency to form blood clots, inflammation, high blood pressure, irritation of the digestive tract, depressed immune function, sterility, cell proliferation, cancer and weight gain,." according to Dr. Enig

For the body to function properly, there should be a 1:1 ratio of omega-6 to omega-3 in the diet. To give you an idea of how much omega-6 is available in the highly processed diet we eat today, non-organic eggs can have an omega-6 to omega-3 ratio of 16:1! With the example of eggs, the feed that is given to chickens is what determines the nutritional content of the eggs. Since conventional chickens can be given a feed with a lot of these cheap oils, the eggs they produce therefore have higher values of deleterious polyunsaturated fats.

Omega-3 Fatty Acids and Thyroid Health

As mentioned in previous chapters, omega-3 supplementation plays a significant role for people with Hashimoto's thyroiditis. Research reveals that it decreases disease activity and can help decrease anti-inflammatory drug intake.[47]

There is also proof that omega-3 fatty acids can help reduce inflammation in the bowel. Therefore, this could be an additional benefit to healing the gut (which is of utmost importance when considering optimal thyroid function).

In direct association with the thyroid, there has been a study performed that looked at the synergistic effect of DHA and T3. The study suggested that DHA present inside of the cell enhanced the fat-burning potential of the thyroid hormone T3.[49] Obviously, more research needs to be done in order to confirm this, but it shows promise for incorporating fish oils or fatty fish into the diet of a person with hypothyroidism in order to enhance metabolism.

Fish Oil Supplementation

What supplement of fish oil to use is highly debated, and obviously a lot of homework needs to be done by the consumer to make sure that the fish oils one takes is safe, bio-available, sustainable and contains the right amount of DHA/EPA. In general, one can ask the manufacturer for a certificate of analysis (COA). This shows the levels of ingredients and heavy metals found in a product by a third-party lab. If the manufacturer is not willing to give you this, there is reason to suspect that a product is not trustworthy. You can also check to see if the product is supported by IFOS, the International Fish Oil Standards (IFOS) Program which is a third-party testing and certification program for fish oils.

It should be noted that the less processed a fish oil is, the better it will be absorbed by the body. As far as the thyroid is concerned, it looks like DHA may be more important to consider. You may need one to three grams of DHA per day in order to enhance thyroid function. Of course this varies for each person, but this is a good place to start. (There are other sources that recommend up to ten grams per day, but this seems extreme and there is not a lot of research to back it up.).

Remember that eating wild fish is also very beneficial despite the concerns about polychlorinated biphenyl (PCB), dioxins and other heavy metals that might be found in them. This is because seafood also contains good amounts of selenium which binds with heavy metals and removes them from the body. Smaller fish have less risk of heavy metal contamination, so choosing fish and fish oils from fish like anchovies and sardines may be safer.

Liver oils like cod liver oil have lower amounts of EPA and DHA but also have higher concentrations of important vitamins like A, D, and K2, all of which are vital for thyroid health. Of course each individual is different, but for general overall health, this may be a better choice.

Saturated Fats and the Thyroid

Saturated fats, especially from medium-chain triglycerides, benefit metabolism and the optimal functioning of the thyroid gland. We have discussed the many functions that saturated fats are responsible for in the body. It is important to note, however, that you should not be getting saturated fats from conventional meat and dairy. These fats are corroded, as they are filled with toxins, hormones and antibiotics. Always choose organic meat and dairy (if tolerated).

Different Therapeutic Diets to Consider for Hypothyroidism

Specific Carbohydrate Diet (SCD)

The specific carbohydrate diet was created in order to address certain inflammatory bowel diseases such as ulcerative colitis, Crohn's disease, celiac disease, diverticulitis, cystic fibrosis, and chronic diarrhea.

It is based on the fact that specific "bad" bacteria feed on disaccharides and polysaccharides to produce inflammation and therefore exacerbate the intestinal diseases mentioned above. The diet works on excluding complex carbohydrates and therefore starving the bacteria that cause inflammation.

In a recent clinical study that looked at the efficacy of the SCD diet on active ulcerative colitis and Crohn's disease in twenty-six patients at Seattle Children's Hospital IBD Center, the SCD diet was able to put the diseases into remission.[50] Of course, more large-scale studies need to be done in order to support this evidence, but, it certainly looks promising.

FODMAPS

FODMAP is an acronym that stands for Fermentable Oligosaccharides, Disaccharides, Monosaccharides and Polyols. In plain English, they are a group of carbohydrates that are poorly absorbed in the small intestine and are fermented in the small and large intestine.

Oligosaccharides

Oligosaccharides are found in gluten-containing foods like wheat, rye, and barley; vegetables like onion, garlic, artichokes, leeks, beetroot, and cabbage; fruits such as watermelon, peaches, prunes, nectarines and most dried fruit; and legumes like red kidney beans, soya beans and baked beans.

Disaccharides

Disaccharides are found in any dairy product containing lactose.

Monosaccharides

Monosaccharides are found in fruits like apples, pears, watermelon, mangos, cherries, and boysenberries; fruit juice from high-fructose fruits; honey; sweeteners such as high-fructose corn syrup; and vegetables such as asparagus and snap peas.

Polyols

Polyols are sugar alcohols found in sorbitol and mannitol; fruits like apples, pears, avocados, apricots, peaches, plums, prunes and watermelon; and vegetables such as sweet potato, cauliflower, mushrooms and snap peas.

If you decide to follow a low FODMAPs diet, then you will need to exclude the above list from your existing diet.

Foods to Include on a Low-FODMAPs Diet

Foods that you can include are listed below:

Grains: Gluten-free flours, quinoa, buckwheat

Fruits: Bananas, most berries, grapes, lemons, limes, mandarin oranges, kiwis, pineapple, passion fruit, rhubarb, honeydew and melon

Vegetables: Bok choy, green beans, parsnips, silverbeets, cucumbers, carrots, celery, eggplant, lettuce, potatoes, yams, tomatoes and zucchini

Sweeteners: Maple syrup

In a recent review looking at the efficacy of a low-FODMAPs diet in decreasing gastrointestinal symptoms associated with IBS, the literature indicated that restriction of FODMAPs is an effective dietary intervention for reducing IBS symptoms.[52]

It is important to note that every individual is unique and not all foods listed as FODMAPs will produce negative outcomes. More research needs to be done in order to assess the safety of long-term adherence to a low-FODMAPs diet.

It is important to discuss a low-FODMAPs diet with your doctor, as many people with thyroid conditions also suffer from IBS. Because there is a link between intestinal health and autoimmune thyroid disease, maintaining a healthy gastrointestinal tract is necessary. If you are a thyroid patient who has been diagnosed with IBS or SIBO (small intestinal bacterial overgrowth), combining the FODMAPs diet with the autoimmune protocol diet (discussed later) may help.

Paleo and Autoimmune Protocol Diet

My experience with thyroid patients over the years has led me to recommend diets similar to the Paleo and autoimmune protocol (AIP) diet. It is important to understand what they are and how they are different in order to implement a meal plan that works specifically for you and your needs as a thyroid patient.

The standard Paleolithic diet's philosophy is to eat in accordance with how our ancestors ate in order to enhance optimal health. I'm not sure I can justify this claim with science, however, I have already outlined some of the more "dangerous" foods for the thyroid such as gluten and dairy which are omitted from the Paleo diet.

Below are foods that are typically not allowed on a Paleo diet:

- Cereal grains
- Legumes (including peanuts)
- Dairy
- Refined sugar
- Potatoes
- Processed foods
- Salt
- Refined vegetable oils

Below are foods that are allowed on a Paleo diet:

- Grass-fed meats and poultry
- Fish/Seafood
- Fresh fruits and veggies
- Eggs
- Nuts and seeds
- Oils like olive, avocado and coconut (walnut, flaxseed and macadamia are also allowed)

In general, for many patients with thyroid disease, eating in a way similar to what is outlined here helps them to increase their energy levels, decrease brain fog, decrease inflammation (associated with things like arthritis, joint pain, or muscle aches) and to lose weight.

A 2015 review in the *American Journal of Clinical Nutrition* looked at the effect of a Paleo diet in relation to patients with metabolic syndrome (certain conditions that increase one's risk for cardiovascular disease and stroke like a large waistline and high blood pressure, cholesterol and triglycerides). It showed that there were greater short-term improvements in metabolic syndrome components (lowered cholesterol, triglycerides and blood pressure and a reduced waistline) on a Paleo diet as compared to guideline-based control diets.[54]

This is good news for people with thyroid disease because metabolic syndrome is associated with thyroid disease.

In my experience, many people see an improvement in symptoms such as bloating, insomnia, fatigue, brain fog and constipation on a Paleo protocol. However, for many others, a more strict approach may need to be implemented. The autoimmune protocol (AIP) is a version of the Paleo diet that, in addition to excluding grains and dairy, also excludes eggs, nuts and seeds and their oils and nightshade vegetables. Once people start to feel better, they can reintroduce these foods in moderation but in general should stick to a Paleo lifestyle.

The Autoimmune Protocol (AIP)

Below is a simple run-down of how to apply an autoimmune protocol:

Food Group	Avoid	Eat
Meats and Seafood	Conventional meat and poultry, farmed raised seafood	Organic and grass-fed beef, bison, chicken, turkey, boar, wild-caught fish and seafood, game meats, bone broth

Grains	All gluten from wheat, rye and barley, oats, rice, millet, quinoa, buckwheat	None
Legumes	Most beans, soy/edamame, peanuts	Snap peas, string beans, haricot vert
Vegetables	Nightshades like eggplants, tomatoes, onions, white potatoes, Goji berries and all pepper based spices like cayenne, nutmeg and paprika	Everything else including asparagus, Brussels sprouts, cabbage, leafy greens, broccoli, cauliflower, cucumbers, beets, squash, carrots, sweet potatoes
Fruit	None	All fruits are permitted, but not exceed two to five fruits per day. (Stay below 20 grams of fructose.)
Dairy	Cheese, yogurt, ghee, butter, ice cream, half and half	Coconut milk

Eggs	All kinds	None
Nuts and Seeds	Almonds, cacao, coffee cashews, macadamias, sunflower seeds, pumpkin seeds, chia seeds, sesame seeds	None
Fermented Foods	Fermented soy products	Kombucha, sauerkraut, kimchi, kefir made with water or coconut water
Sugar and Sugar Replacement	All types of sugar like sugar, high fructose corn syrup, coconut sugar, date sugar, corn sugar, stevia, agave, molasses, honey, maple syrup	None
Fats	All butter and ghee, all margarines, canola oil and all other seed oils	Avocado, avocado oil, Coconut oil, Olive oil, lard, fat

Food Additives	Carrageenan, guar gum,aspartame, benzoic acid, MSG, sulfates/sulfites, nitrates, nitrites	None
Alcohol	Beer, wine, liquor and sugar extracts like vanilla extract	None

Why Nuts, Seeds, Nightshade Vegetables, and Eggs Are Not Allowed on an Autoimmune Protocol

Lectins.

Approximately 30 percent of the food we eat contains lectins, which are carbohydrate-binding proteins. Because of these binding properties, they can cause nutrient deficiencies and can cause severe intestinal distress in sensitive individuals. These symptoms can lead to increased intestinal permeability, which is linked to autoimmune disease.

Just like gluten can cause an autoimmune attack by means of cross-reactivity (in other words, your body confuses gluten with a dangerous bacteria and attacks it and other tissues that resemble it), in sensitive people, lectin can do the same.

Research shows that decreasing lectins in certain individuals can decrease symptoms associated with an autoimmune disease.[56]

Lectins can be divided into two sub-types called prolamines and agglutanins. Prolamins are storage proteins in plants and account for half of the total protein in plants. The most well-known prolamine is gliadin (a part of the gluten protein), found in wheat. Other examples are hordein (found in barley), secalin (found in rye), orzenin (found in rice) and avenin (found in oats).

The problem with prolamins is that they are not sufficiently broken down into amino acids by human enzymes. These larger proteins therefore have the ability to travel down the intestinal tract intact, and can cause leaky gut and cross over to the blood, stimulating an autoimmune attack.

Agglutanins are another form of lectins that have the ability to clump together red blood cells. These proteins protect seeds from fungal infection as well as from predators like insects. An interesting fact is that genetically modified grains have higher levels of agglutanins to help protect against insects. They are so effective, in fact, that the gene for wheat germ agglutinin has been added to genetically modified corn.

Like prolamins, agglutanins can cause increased intestinal

permeability and can stimulate an autoimmune response. To give you a good example of the extent to which an agglutinin can throw off the immune system, the agglutinin found in tomatoes is being studied for its use as an adjuvant (an immune-stimulating chemical) in vaccines because it activates antibody production. (Ok, I am not saying that everyone has to stop eating tomatoes, but in sensitive individuals, tomatoes can increase a leaky gut and therefore an autoimmune response.)

Although lectins found in grains, legumes and pseudo-grains will not make us sick right away, they do have the ability to cause disease with years of consumption. Especially when considering an autoimmune condition, lectins in all food sources should be avoided until symptoms resolve.

Foods that contain lectins and should be avoided:

Grains	Pseudo-grains	Legumes
• Wheat (including einkorn, durum and semolina) • Rye & barley • Corn • Kamut • Millet • Oats • Rice • Sorghum • Spelt • Triticale • Wild rice	• Amaranth • Buckwheat • Chia • Quinoa	• Alfalfa • Carob • Chickpea • Clover • Common bean • Fava bean • Field or garden pea • Lentil • Lima Bean • Mesquite • Mung bean • Peanut • Pigeon pea • Rooibos • Runner Bean • Soybean

Digestive enzyme inhibitors and phytic acid and phytates.

Digestive enzyme inhibitors decrease the ability of pancreatic enzymes to break food down. They prevent the enzymes that take apart proteins and carbohydrates. They are predominantly found in grains, pseudo-grains, legumes, and seeds. If a seed requires chewing before ingestion or it is ground into a flour, digestive enzyme inhibitors are released into the gut and can cause increased intestinal permeability as well as gut dysbiosis (both very common issues with autoimmune thyroiditis). Digestive enzyme inhibitors also increase the production of pancreatic enzymes which use up amino acids and deplete nutrients from the body.

Phytic acid and phytates are other anti-nutrients that decrease the ability of digestive enzymes and increase gut permeability.

In addition to grains, pseudo-grains, and legumes, it is important to avoid nuts and seeds and their oils for the reasons listed here. Following is a list of nuts and seeds to avoid when following an autoimmune protocol:

Nuts and Seeds to Avoid on an AIP diet:

Nuts and oils	Seeds and oils
• Almonds	• Chia
• Brazil nuts	• Flaxseed
• Cashews	• Hemp seeds
• Chestnuts	• Poppy
• Hazelnuts	• Pumpkin
• Macadamia nuts	• Sesame
• Pecans	• Sunflower
• Pine nuts	
• Pistachios	
• Walnuts	

Saponins: alkaloids and glycoalkaloids.

Saponins are anti-nutrients that act like a detergent, increasing intestinal permeability and stimulating antibody production. Depending on their size, saponins can have either a toxic or a beneficial effect on the intestine. The toxic saponins, also known as glycoalkaloids, can create holes in enterocytes (the cells the intestine) and can actually cause damage to these cells. These types of saponins are found in night-shade vegetables. Researchers have hypothesized that moderate consumption of nightshade vegetables can contribute to autoimmune disease.

Following is a list of night shade vegetables you should avoid:

Nightshade Vegetables and Plants

- Ashwaganda
- Bell peppers
- Bush tomatoes
- Cape gooseberries
- Cocona
- Eggplant
- Garden huckleberries
- Goji berries
- Hot peppers
- Kutjera
- Naranjillas
- Paprika
- Pepinos
- Pimentos
- Potatoes (sweet potatoes are ok)
- Tamarillos
- Tomatillos
- Tomatoes

Lysozyme.

Lysozyme is an enzyme found in egg whites that breaks down cell membrane components of gram-negative bacteria and transports these bacteria across the gut into the blood. This can stimulate an autoimmune attack and is the reason why eggs should be avoided on an autoimmune protocol. However, once the gut is healed, eggs can be reintroduced in moderation to the diet.

A note on insoluble fiber.

Many people worry about irritating their intestines further by adding more raw vegetables to their diet. Increased soluble fiber in the diet helps to protect against cardiovascular disease and cancer, improves insulin sensitivity, and helps to remove toxins from the body. If you initially cannot handle a lot of fiber, add supplements in the form of plant enzymes or cook all of your vegetables initially until gut inflammation improves.

Beware of histamines.

Histamine is a type of molecule that is detoxified by gut enzymes. However, if there are not enough of these enzymes available in the gut (which is usually the case with people who have SIBO or a leaky gut), histamines are not detoxified and can accumulate within the body. Histamine intolerance is more likely if you have a thyroid condition or are taking thyroid hormone replacement drugs.

Symptoms of histamine intolerance (that usually happen shortly after histamine-containing foods are ingested) can include:

- Diarrhea
- Headache
- Sinus symptoms
- Itchy or watery eyes
- Asthma
- Low blood pressure
- Arrhythmia
- Hives, rashes and flushing

Foods that contain high levels of histamines include fish that is not appropriately handled and cooled after fishing, processed and fermented meats, cheeses, fermented vegetables, soy products and alcoholic beverages.

Fermented vegetables can be a good source of probiotics, but they may not be tolerated at the beginning of your journey to healing your gut and reversing thyroid symptoms as they may contain high levels of histamines. The best way to understand if you have a histamine intolerance is to keep a food journal and document if you experience any of the afore-mentioned symptoms after consuming a histamine-containing food.

For a more in-depth look at the autoimmune protocol, take a look at Dr. Sarah Ballantyne's book, *The Paleo Approach: Reverse Autoimmune Diseases and Heal Your Body.*

Important Nutrients for Thyroid Disease

In this chapter I address the vitamins and minerals that are essential to thyroid function and overall health. After reading this, you will appreciate the importance of eating a varied diet and will have a better understanding of which foods are essential to include in a daily meal plan for thyroid health.

Although I would like to think that people can get all of the nutrition they need to heal from diet alone, my clinical and personal experiences have proven otherwise. It is my professional opinion that supplements are necessary and should serve as a welcome addition to an already healthy and diversified diet. Please note, however, that not all supplements are created equal. I will discuss what to look for in a supplement in this chapter.

Magnesium

Magnesium is a mineral that is found in all living things, including humans. It is involved with over three hundred biochemical reactions in the body. It serves as an important cofactor to enzyme regulation, it is essential in the production of glutathione (the body's most powerful antioxidant), it is involved in the production of energy, it regulates and maintains the body's internal instructions for building proteins and new cells (in other words, our DNA) and it balances other minerals such as potassium, calcium, and sodium.

Since magnesium is vital for the proper functioning of the body's cells, it is definitely a mineral that could prevent the body from performing optimally when deficient. Low magnesium status is implicated in hypertension, coronary heart disease, type 2 diabetes, and metabolic syndrome.

Magnesium Deficiency Is on the Rise

According to the World Health Organization (WHO), magnesium deficiency is common in the United States and other Westernized countries. In the United States alone, 75 percent of the population does not meet the Recommended Daily Intake of magnesium. In fact, magnesium consumption has decreased by more than half as compared to a century ago.

In France, one study found that over 70 percent of men and nearly 80 percent of women have a magnesium deficiency.

In Finland the government was so convinced of how important magnesium was to heart health that they implemented a campaign to increase magnesium intake via magnesium salt substitutes. Finland's death rates due to heart-related issues fell from number one to number ten.

It is possible that one of the reasons that magnesium deficiency is not more widely recognized is because there aren't accurate and inexpensive tests that can be used to diagnose it. However, the good news is that one can supplement with magnesium or eat more magnesium-rich foods without any side effects to see if certain symptoms associated with magnesium deficiency improve.

Why Is Magnesium Deficiency More Prevalent Today?

There has been an ongoing theme in this book that eating real, whole foods is of utmost importance. Therefore, it should come as no surprise that with the increase of processed and refined foods in our diets, there has also been an increase in vitamin and mineral deficiencies.

Magnesium is typically found in whole grains, nuts, beans, meat, dairy, and green leafy vegetables. These common foods, aside from being genetically modified or pesticide laden, have been stripped of their nutrient density and magnesium content through processing.

A study in *Nutrition and Health* found consistent declines in magnesium content of food through the years in the United Kingdom. Between the years of 1940 and 1991, the magnesium content of vegetables, fruits, meats and cheeses declined by 24 percent, 17 percent, 15 percent and 26 percent, respectively.[61]

Also note that magnesium content varies greatly depending on agricultural practices, the quality of the soil, and storage and transportation methods.

In addition to the above, most people do not make it a habit to include abundant fruits, vegetables, nuts, and seeds into their daily diet, and instead eat a diet predominantly made up of processed and refined white sugar and flour. This obviously enhances one's chances of developing a magnesium deficiency.

Another interesting fact is that no current regulations require testing or monitoring of nutritional content of produce or meat sources. Therefore, it's anyone's guess how much magnesium is available from food.

What Are Some Symptoms of Magnesium Deficiency:

Symptoms of magnesium deficiency are quite general and can be mistaken for another chronic disease such as hypothyroidism.

Conditions related to chronic magnesium deficiency include the following:

- Depression
- Chronic fatigue syndrome
- ADHD
- Epilepsy
- Parkinson's disease
- Sleep problems
- Migraine
- Cluster headaches
- Osteoporosis
- Premenstrual syndrome
- Chest pain (angina)
- Cardiac arrhythmias
- Coronary artery disease and atherosclerosis
- Hypertension
- Type 2 diabetes
- Asthma

Magnesium and Hypothyroidism

People with hypothyroidism tend to have consistent underlying inflammation that can increase levels of C-reactive protein, or CRP, in the body. (CRP is a marker of inflammation.) Magnesium can lower CRP by decreasing inflammation within the body. Therefore, many symptoms associated with magnesium deficiency and hypothyroidism (for example, feeling tired all the time) can be alleviated.

A recent animal study showed that signs of inflammation in hypothyroid rats were markedly improved when their diets were supplemented with thyroxine and magnesium as opposed to thyroxine alone.[63]

As mentioned previously, blood glucose control is imperative in those suffering from hypothyroidism. A review and meta-analysis of randomized controlled trials on the effect of magnesium on insulin sensitivity and blood glucose control found that supplementation with magnesium for more than four months showed clear improvement in fasting glucose in both diabetic and non-diabetic subjects.[64] In plain English, taking magnesium can help one to regulate blood sugar levels.

What Should I Include in My Diet to Boost My Magnesium Levels:

Now that we are all convinced of how important magnesium is, let's get to the practical stuff. Including magnesium-rich foods as well as supplementing with magnesium are important to improve a deficiency and to support optimal health.

How Much Magnesium Do I Need for Optimal Health?

The current American Recommended Daily Allowance (RDA) for magnesium is 6 milligrams per 1 kilogram of body weight. In other words, if you weigh 60 kilograms, you would need 360 milligrams of magnesium per day. The RDA was created by the government to cover what one would need in order to prevent major deficiencies, but it falls short of boosting the body's performance to optimal and functional health. Therefore, many experts recommend an increase of the RDA as they suggest that at least 300 milligrams per day are needed simply to cover what is lost on a daily basis. People who deal with stressful situations, are ill, or engage in exercise have even higher magnesium requirements.

As thyroid disease causes inflammation, and magnesium is proven to decrease inflammation, aiming for six to eight milligrams per kilogram per day may be your best bet. You may need more, depending on stress and training levels. Of course, it goes without saying that you should work with your doctor, functional medicine practitioner, or nutritionist to find the ideal dosage for you.

For more information on what types of magnesium tests are available for a more accurate diagnosis of magnesium deficiency , please refer to *The Magnesium Miracle* by Dr. Carolyn Dean.

Which Foods Are Rich in Magnesium?

If you want to have a diet rich in magnesium, it is important to eat foods such as green vegetables, nuts, seeds, legumes and unprocessed grains on a daily basis. Remember, however, that people with hypothyroidism should remain gluten-free and this creates one less important source of magnesium from most grains. In addition to this, grains, legumes, nuts, and seeds have an anti nutrient called phytic acid, which decreases the absorption of magnesium and can exacerbate a leaky gut. If you have decreased levels of stomach acid, an inflamed intestine or other chronic ailments of the intestine, eating raw foods, nuts, and seeds may exacerbate your problem. Therefore, until the gut is healed, it is definitely warranted to take a magnesium supplement to make up for what cannot be absorbed.

Following are some foods that are better sources of magnesium for anyone following an autoimmune paleo protocol:

Some Paleo Foods That Are Rich in Magnesium:

Figs	Avocado	Caviar
Apricots	Coconut meat	Raisins
Dates	Collard greens	Sweet potato
Prunes	Snails	Dandelion greens

Supplementing with Magnesium

According to Dr. Dean, author of *The Magnesium Miracle*, the most absorbable form of magnesium is magnesium citrate. You can find this in powder form and add it to water for optimal absorption. However, magnesium citrate can have a laxative effect and should be avoided in people who already have looser stools. For this group of people, magnesium in the form of magnesium taurate, glycinate, or orotate are recommended.

If oral magnesium causes too many loose stools, you can opt for magnesium oil, which is basically supersaturated magnesium chloride in water. Dr. Norman Shealy, M.D., Ph.D., neurosurgeon, and world-renowned pain management expert, recommends using a 25 percent solution spray of magnesium oil per day and claims that any magnesium deficiency can be corrected within four to six weeks.

When Should I Take Magnesium Supplements?

The best time to take magnesium is in the morning and in the evening. If you use the oil, spray the oil on your legs and arms before bedtime. (If it produces a tingling sensation, you may need to dilute the magnesium oil in some water in order to decrease the dose. Also, if you feel itchy after applying the oil, it is absorbed within thirty minutes, so after this time frame, feel free to wash it off.)

209

Zinc

Zinc is a vital mineral that is involved in over two hundred different enzyme reactions within the body. It has a variety of roles, which include gene expression and communication between cells, detoxification, protein production, collagen production, immune function and thyroid function.

Zinc is a necessary component for converting T4 (the storage form of thyroid hormone) into T3 (the active form of thyroid hormone used in the cells). Zinc is also needed to form TSH (thyroid stimulating hormone) and can be depleted when TSH is consistently being produced in high levels when one is hypothyroid. Conversely, thyroid hormones are essential for the absorption of zinc.

For this reason, most people with hypothyroidism are, in fact, zinc deficient and need to correct the deficiency by eating zinc-rich foods as well as with supplementation.

Signs of Zinc Deficiency

- Poor neurological function
- Weak immunity
- Diarrhea
- Frequent allergies
- Thinning hair

- Acne or rashes

Zinc Deficiency and Hair Loss

For many of you out there suffering with hypothyroidism, you may be appalled by how much hair is lost on a daily basis. Hair loss is an unfortunate symptom of hypothyroidism. What most people do not know is that in addition to needing sufficient iron stores as well as thyroid hormones to support hair growth, people also need zinc to maintain a healthy head of hair.

In a case report from 2013 looking at a twenty-eight year old woman with severe hair loss and asymptomatic scaly lesions on her scalp (as well as other hypothyroid symptoms), treating her with thyroxine alone did not reverse the hair loss. When 50 milligrams of elemental zinc was given twice per day in addition to the thyroxine, within a month, the scaly lesions were gone, and complete re-growth of the hair was seen within four months.[65]

In another case study of a four-year-old girl with severe hair loss and no other symptoms or medical issues, supplementing with 50 milligrams of zinc every day stopped the hair loss in three weeks.[66]

As someone who suffered from a lot of hair loss for most of my adult life, I can say that I was relieved to find this piece of information. I supplemented with zinc and my hair stopped

211

falling out!

How Much Zinc Do I Need for Optimal Health?

The Recommended Daily Allowance (RDA) for zinc is 11 milligrams per day for adult men and 8 milligrams per day for adult women. Obviously, this amount does not even come close to the doses that we have seen to support optimal hair growth (let alone thyroid function).

In the presence of a deficiency, 50 milligrams of elemental zinc (from 220 milligrams of zinc sulphate) can be taken twice daily for three months to stop hair loss. As always, work with your health care practitioner to find the right dosage for you.

Which Foods Are Rich in Zinc?

Once again, I hate to disappoint my vegan/vegetarian audience, however, the research shows that the phytic acid found in grains, legumes, nuts, and seeds inhibits zinc absorption. It is also easier to extract zinc from meat than from non-meat sources. Therefore, following a Paleo dietary protocol is more conducive to absorbing an optimal amount of zinc.

Paleo Foods Rich in Zinc

Oysters	Beef	Liver
Crab	Pork	Lamb
Lobsters	Chicken	Veal

Zinc Supplementation

When looking for a good zinc supplement, keep in mind that research shows that zinc gluconate, acetate, citrate or sulphate are acceptable forms of zinc.[68] Remember that each zinc compound contains a specific amount of elemental zinc, which is what you want to be taking. In general, the label always lists the amount of elemental zinc the supplement contains, so you do not have to worry about calculating it yourself.

Copper

Copper is zinc's partner in crime. Both are needed for gene expression, bone formation, immune support and collagen formation. Dietary copper is also important in resistance to infection. If you take too much zinc, copper depletion may occur, and therefore, when taking zinc, it is important to take copper as well. In general, it is recommended that you take 1 milligram of copper for every 15 milligrams of zinc.

Signs of Copper Deficiency

- Fatigue
- Arthritis
- Osteoporosis
- Paleness
- Low body temperature, or always feeling cold
- Anemia
- Brittle bones
- Frequently getting sick
- Muscle soreness
- Joint pain
- A stunt in growth
- Hair thinning or balding
- Unexplained weight loss
- Bruising
- Skin inflammation and sores

Copper and Hypothyroidism

Copper, in cooperation with other minerals, like zinc, potassium and calcium, help to balance thyroid function. A deficit or too much of any of these minerals, could stop the thyroid from working properly.

Copper also plays a role in proper absorption and storage of iron. If there is a copper deficiency, iron-deficient anemia can occur, further exacerbating common symptoms of hypothyroidism such as fatigue and hair loss. Copper is also responsible for the formation of melanin and therefore plays a role in the pigmentation of hair, skin, and nails.

In a recent study performed with children with congenital hypothyroidism, a positive correlation was found between thyroid hormone levels and copper.[69] In other words, when thyroid hormones are low, copper levels are low, and vice versa. Although bigger studies need to be performed to confirm this finding, the study suggested that severely hypothyroid children are at risk of developing a copper deficiency. In other words, a sufficient copper level in people with hypothyroidism is necessary for optimal health. Also, as you can see from the list of symptoms of copper deficiency, many, such as feeling cold or losing hair, are also symptoms of hypothyroidism.

How Much Copper Is Needed for Optimal Health?

The Recommended Daily Allowance (RDA) for copper for adults is 900 micrograms per day. As stated earlier, if you have a zinc deficiency and are trying to correct for this, 1 milligram of copper should be taken for every 15 milligrams of zinc. There is not enough evidence to suggest an ideal amount of copper to sustain optimal health or to prevent disease.

Which Foods Contain Copper?

Foods that are rich in zinc are generally rich in copper as well. (Isn't nature wonderful?) So, please refer to the list of foods that are rich in zinc to see which ones are rich in copper. (Copper is also found in cocoa powder, kale, shitake mushrooms and tomatoes.) You can also obtain copper from cooking in cast iron pots and pans. Some of the copper is absorbed into the food that you cook in the pots and pans.

Copper Supplementation

In general, 1.5 to 3 grams of copper per day are ideal for supplementation. Copper can easily be obtained from the diet. However, if you do decide to supplement with it, copper is available in the following forms: cupric oxide, copper gluconate and copper sulphate.

Selenium

In my humble opinion, selenium is the king mineral when it comes to thyroid health. The thyroid gland actually contains the highest amount of selenium in the body, as compared to any other organ. Selenium is needed to create glutathione (the body's master antioxidant) and other selenoproteins (proteins that have selenium attached to them) that contribute to balancing iodine metabolism (and decreasing inflammation) when thyroid hormones are created. It is a wonderful ingredient in terms of helping the liver to detoxify the body, helping support thyroid health once again. Selenium is also a vital mineral that helps convert T4 to T3, which is actively used in our cells.

Signs of Selenium Deficiency

- Thyroid dysfunction
- Weakened immune system
- Infertility in men and women
- Depression
- Heart disease
- Increased risk of cancer

Selenium and Hashimoto's Thyroiditis

When it comes to Hashimoto's thyroiditis, selenium can help to decrease antibodies as well as to decrease the inflammation by balancing T cell activity, decreasing cytokine activity and decreasing thyroid cell destruction. Studies from several countries have confirmed that an increased selenium intake is associated with a decrease in Hashimoto's thyroiditis.[71]

It is important to mention here that selenium and iodine work together. There are studies that suggest that excessive iodine can perpetuate an autoimmune attack; however, it seems that this is the case only if one is deficient in selenium. Conversely, if one gets too much selenium and is iodine deficient, this could also aggravate a thyroid condition.[72,73] (More on iodine later.)

How Much Selenium Is Needed for Optimal Thyroid Function?

The Recommended Daily Allowance for selenium is 55 micrograms per day. However, this is not enough to reduce thyroid antibodies. The lowest dose established by studies to reduce thyroid antibodies is 200 micrograms per day.[74] (Even 100 micrograms per day was not enough.) Selenium should be taken together with vitamin E on an empty stomach to ensure proper absorption.

The consequences of high-dose selenium intake over a long period time are not yet known, and therefore it is important to stick to a dose of 200 micrograms per day for no more than three months. After this time period, antibodies should be checked to confirm a decrease.

Paleo Foods Rich in Selenium

Yellowfin tuna	Grass-fed beef	Chicken
Cooked halibut	Turkey	Free-range eggs
Sardines	Beef liver	Spinach

Here, it's prudent to mention that although Brazil nuts are known for having a high selenium content, there are two reasons not to eat them when you have hypothyroidism. First, as mentioned previously, Brazil nuts contain phytic acid, which blocks the absorption of selenium, and second, the quantity of selenium in the nuts is dependent on the soil in which the nuts are grown. Therefore, one can get varying amounts of selenium from Brazil nuts depending on where they originated.

Selenium Supplementation

Selenium can be found in the form of selenomethionine or sodium selenite. Not many studies have been performed to assess which is better absorbed by the body, however, one study showed that selenomethionine was better absorbed.[75]

Iodine: Does It Help or Does It Hurt?

Iodine is a trace element that is needed to create thyroid hormones. If there is excessive iodine present, there is more cell death in the thyroid. The reason for this is that hydrogen peroxide is produced when iodine is converted into its usable form. If there is insufficient selenium or glutathione present to clear the hydrogen peroxide, it builds up within the thyroid tissue causing cell death and inflammation.

Although the above is true, iodine is a highly debated nutrient within the hypothyroidism world, as there are many practitioners who swear by big doses of iodine for optimal health. However, when it comes to autoimmunity, it is my opinion that iodine supplementation should be undertaken with caution.

The irony of the situation is that if one does have an iodine deficiency, this causes a goiter, which means that the thyroid gland increases in size in order to absorb more iodine from the blood. Iodine deficiency related to goiters is so common worldwide that governments of various countries have corrected for this deficiency by adding iodine to the food supply. However, studies have shown that in countries where iodine was added to the food supply, iodine deficiency decreased and Hashimoto's thyroiditis increased.

Two cross-sectional population studies performed in Denmark measured thyroid antibodies before and after the implementation of adding iodine to salt. After five years, an increase in the prevalence of thyroid antibodies was seen.[76]

Another study of 1,085 participants in Sao Paulo showed a 17 percent increase in autoimmune thyroiditis over a five year period.[77]

The above information gives me reason to believe that iodine is one of those nutrients that too little or too much of is not good for optimal health. I do believe in eating foods that contain iodine within the context of a Paleo diet, but, I would not supplement with iodine unless proper testing was undertaken to determine a true iodine deficiency.

How Much Iodine Is Sufficient?

The Recommended Daily Allowance for iodine is 150 micrograms per day for adults. Eating more iodine than this could definitely enhance one's susceptibility to inflammation and an autoimmune attack. In the typical Western diet alone, one could easily get this amount of iodine before lunch because processed, conventional foods like dairy and wheat products have increased iodine, either due to the feed of the animals or due to the supplementation of processed foods with iodine. Also, processed foods are laden with salt, which is also typically enriched with iodine.

Paleo Foods Rich in Iodine

Haddock	Sea vegetables	Squid
Lobster	Crab	Cod
Cod	Broth	Mackerel

The autoimmune protocol for helping balance the immune system recommends plenty of seafood, which is, in fact, iodine rich. This should be the main source of iodine within the diet. As excess iodine seems to be affected by whether or not there is a selenium deficiency, you should work with your doctor to correct for any deficiencies before eating a lot of seafood.

Halogens and Iodine

The subject of iodine becomes even more gray when looking at halogens such as chlorine, bromine and fluorine. These metals bind with receptor sites within the body that are usually designated for iodine. If they are present in excess quantities, they interrupt the absorption, metabolism, distribution or excretion of iodine and can lead to iodine toxicity, even at therapeutic amounts. Again, it is important to work with your health care practitioner to test for these issues before consuming iodine-rich foods.

Iron/Ferritin

Iron is a vital part of hemoglobin, the protein structure in the body that carries oxygen from the lungs to every cell in the body. It is the iron itself that binds to the oxygen. Ferritin, the body's reserve protein for iron, is responsible for the transport of T3 to the cell nucleus as well as for the utilization of T3 hormone. Therefore, iron is an integral part of optimal thyroid function.

Symptoms of Low Iron Status:

- Fatigue
- Difficulty concentrating
- Decreased immune function
- Hair loss
- Pale skin
- Weakness
- Shortness of breath
- Headache
- Dizziness and light-headedness
- Fast heartbeat
- Poor appetite

Once again we see that symptoms of iron deficiency coincide with symptoms of hypothyroidism. Therefore, anyone with hypothyroidism should definitely test for iron deficiency, specifically from ferritin stores.

Ferritin and Hair Loss

When the body is low in iron, it uses the iron for more important processes in the body (like breathing) and takes it away from less important ones (like hair growth). Thinning hair is not only caused by a zinc deficiency but also by insufficient stores of iron. Ferritin levels of 40 ng/mL are required to stop hair loss, 70 ng/ml is required for hair growth, and 90 to 110 ng/ml is needed for optimal thyroid function.

Iron and Thyroid Autoimmunity

Low iron status also seems to increase thyroid antibodies and exacerbates Hashimoto's thyroiditis.

A recent cross-sectional study of 1900 pregnant women was done in order to assess the prevalence of thyroid autoimmunity with iron deficiency. Iron deficiency was defined as a ferritin level of less than 15 mcg/L, thyroid autoimmunity was defined as TPO antibodies of greater than 60 kIU/L and subclinical hypothyroidism was defined as a TSH greater than 2.5 IU/L. The researchers found that iron was inversely correlated with serum TSH levels and positively correlated with free T4 levels. In other words, when iron was low, TSH levels were higher and free T4 levels were lower. Iron deficiency during the first trimester of pregnancy was therefore correlated with a higher prevalence of autoimmune thyroiditis.[79]

Anemia is common in many with Hashimoto's, as this population typically produces low amounts of stomach acid, which hinders the proper absorption of iron. In a 2016 large population-based study done in Europe, there was a correlation between iron deficiency and thyroid disorders.[80]

In my experience, supplementing with extra iron is usually not the way to address low iron status. Following a gluten- and dairy-free diet, taking acid supplements if necessary, and adding nutrient density to the diet are often enough to restore sufficient iron stores. You need to be extremely careful with iron supplementation, as excess iron within the body is very toxic and can be fatal. As always, talk with your doctor to see if iron supplementation is right for you.

The Right Amount of Iron

The Recommended Daily Allowance for iron is 8 milligrams for adult males and 18 milligrams for adult women. The reason women need more is because they lose blood every month with their menstrual cycle. I would not recommend getting more iron than the RDA, as getting sufficient iron is more about absorbing it than actually getting more of it in the diet.

Iron-rich Paleo Foods

Grass-fed beef	Oysters	Coconut milk
Chicken liver	Spinach	
Clams	Coconut meat	

Iron is more readily absorbed from meat sources than from plant sources. However, if you have low levels of stomach acid, adding foods that naturally boost stomach acid production or taking a hydrochloric acid (HCl) supplement will help you to better absorb iron from food.

B Vitamins

Thiamine (Vitamin B1)

Thiamine acts as a coenzyme within the body that works with other B vitamins to produce energy and maintain proper heart and nerve function. It is therefore very important for supporting energy levels and metabolism. It helps to break down carbohydrates, proteins, and fats into glucose (the body's main fuel source). It also helps to form red blood cells, protects the nervous system, boosts immunity, enhances learning and helps maintain a positive mood because it helps the body to withstand stress.

Most of the thiamine we need comes from our diet. However, the bacteria found in the large intestine also produce it.

Some symptoms of thiamine deficiency:

- Anorexia or rapid weight loss
- Poor appetite
- Colitis
- Diarrhea
- Nerve damage
- Fatigue
- Depression or apathy

Thiamine and hypothyroidism.

Although thiamine deficiencies in Westernized countries are rare, there is some preliminary evidence that suggests the useful role of thiamine in reducing fatigue in hypothyroid patients. A few hypothyroid patients given 600 mg of oral thiamine or 100 mg/ml (over 4 days) of parenteral thiamine experienced complete regression of fatigue within a few hours or days. The researchers suggest that there may be a mild thiamine deficiency seen in patients with Hashimoto's due to the dysfunction of the intracellular transport of thiamine or enzymatic abnormalities.[81]

How much thiamine is necessary?

The Recommended Daily Allowance for adults is 1.2 milligrams per day for men and 1.1 milligrams per day for women. There is no evidence of side effects from excess thiamine. Therefore, if you take a B-complex vitamin, in addition to a nutrient-dense diet, this should be sufficient to support optimal health.

Paleo Food Sources of Thiamine

Kiwi	Chicken, lamb, beef, or turkey liver	Asparagus
Ground pork	Yellowfin tuna	Brussel sprouts
Pork tenderloin	Seaweed	

Riboflavin (Vitamin B2)

Riboflavin is another important B vitamin that helps to produce energy and maintain a good metabolism. It acts as an antioxidant and works in conjunction with other B vitamins. In fact, if there is not enough riboflavin available in the diet, other

B vitamins such as folate and vitamin B6 will not do their jobs sufficiently.

Riboflavin has been studied for the prevention of ailments and diseases such as migraine headaches, anemia, cancer, hyperglycemia, hypertension and diabetes.

Signs of riboflavin deficiency.

As with thiamine, riboflavin deficiencies are uncommon in Westernized countries. However, some of the following can be signs of a vitamin B2 deficiency:

- Anemia
- Fatigue
- Nerve damage
- A sluggish metabolism
- Sores or cracks in mouth or on lips
- Skin inflammation and skin disorders, especially around the nose and face
- Increased anxiety and signs of depression

Riboflavin and hypothyroidism.

In people with hypothyroidism, the biochemical pathway that creates active forms of bioflavin for use within the cells is compromised. In other words, without sufficient amounts of thyroid hormone, signs of riboflavin deficiency can be observed, as enough thyroid hormone is needed for riboflavin to function properly. This is important to understand because if you simply take B vitamins and wait for a boost in energy when you do not take any thyroid replacement hormones, you will wait for a long time. Thyroid hormones and B vitamins work together to maintain a healthy metabolism.

Riboflavin and migraine headaches.

Headaches are common for people with hypothyroidism. Many may experience excruciating headaches in the form of a migraine. In a recent review done on riboflavin and migraine headaches, the researchers concluded that riboflavin supplementation can play a positive role in reducing the frequency and the duration of migraine headaches.[85]

Paleo Foods Rich in Riboflavin

Meat and organ meat
Eggs
Green leafy vegetables

Niacin (Vitamin B3)

Niacin is another water-soluble B vitamin that is important to cardiovascular health, particularly in lowering low-density lipoprotein (LDL) or "bad" cholesterol levels as well as in healthy skin formation, brain function, diabetes prevention and joint pain reduction (as it can act as an anti-inflammatory). It has been studied extensively and has been used in high doses to treat various ailments.

There are some initial studies that show that niacin can have side effects or is not tolerated by sensitive people when given in high doses. However, the research is not definitive and most people need not worry about this, as high doses are typically not seen in a B-complex vitamin that is often recommended.

Symptoms of vitamin B3 deficiency.

Niacin deficiency is again very rare in Westernized countries. However, its symptoms can be seen in people who suffer from alcoholism and those who are severely malnourished. Typically, vitamin B deficiency can be defined by dermatitis (skin rash), dementia, and/or diarrhea.

Niacin and hypothyroidism.

There is a bit of debate as to whether or not vitamin B3 is good for people with hypothyroidism. Some research shows that supplementation with niacin decreases total T4 and T3 in the blood. However, there is no change in TSH or free T4. Therefore, the limited research shows that although some thyroid hormones decrease in the blood, a euthyroid (or normal functioning thyroid) state is seen with niacin supplementation. Further research needs to be done in order to make more solid recommendations. In my experience with patients, a B-complex vitamin usually provides the right amount of niacin without any side effects.

Paleo Foods That Are Rich in Niacin

Grass-fed beef	Organ meats	Halibut
Chicken	Anchovies	Mackerel

Pantothenic Acid (Vitamin B5)

Pantothenic acid is a vitamin that is crucial for the functioning of the nervous system. It is also an important coenzyme that helps to manufacture red blood cells as well as sex and stress-related hormones (produced in the adrenal glands). Vitamin B5 is also important in maintaining a healthy digestive tract. It works together with other B vitamins to extract energy from the food we eat.

Symptoms of pantothenic acid deficiency.

A deficiency of this vitamin is uncommon, however, it can be deficient in combination with other B vitamin deficiencies. People at greater risk of a deficiency are alcoholics and women on oral contraceptives. Signs of deficiency include the following:

- Fatigue
- Depression, irritability
- Insomnia
- Upper respiratory infections
- Muscle cramps
- Burning feet
- Vomiting

Pantothenic acid and hypothyroidism.

Vitamin B5 is often used by hypothyroid patients as a way to battle fatigue. However, besides the fact that most people with hypothyroidism have deficiencies in B vitamins, there is no conclusive evidence that demonstrates the effect of pantothenic acid on thyroid function.

Paleo Foods Rich in Pantothenic Acid

Beef liver	Avocado	Duck
Portobello mushrooms	Eggs (if tolerated)	Salmon
Veal	Broccoli	

Pyridoxine (Vitamin B6)

Vitamin B6 is a B vitamin that helps us to produce energy, to produce haemoglobin and to balance blood sugar levels, acts as a natural pain treatment; and boosts immunity. Vitamin B6 is vital to nerve function.

Vitamin B6 deficiency.

Again, this type of deficiency is rare in Westernized countries. However, we are more prone to a vitamin B6 deficiency as we age. Since vitamin B6 is important to nerve function, not getting enough vitamin B6 from one's diet is linked to neuropsychiatric disorders, like seizures, migraines, chronic pain, and depression. Some other symptoms of deficiency are as follows:

- Depression, anxiety
- Confusion
- Muscle pains
- Fatigue
- Worsening PMS symptoms
- Worsening symptoms of anemia

Paleo Foods Rich in Pyridoxine

Turkey breast	Avocado	Chicken breast
Grass-fed beef	Tuna	

Biotin (Vitamin B7)

Biotin is the B vitamin known for hair and nail health. It supports a healthy metabolism, regulates blood sugar (which is also important for hair health) and protects us from cognitive decline.

Biotin deficiency.

Biotin deficiency is rare but can be seen in people who are on anti seizure medication, people who are subject to long-term antibiotic use and people who have digestive issues such as those seen in diseases like Crohn's or Celiac disease (as B7 can be produced by gut bacteria as well). Symptoms can be as follows:

- Dry, irritated skin
- Brittle hair or hair loss
- Chronic fatigue
- Muscle aches and pains
- Nerve damage
- Tingling in the limbs
- Cramps

Biotin and the thyroid.

Here is an interesting fact about biotin that you may not know. In a recent study from the *New England Journal of Medicine,* supplementation with biotin was shown to produce false positives for autoimmune disorders such as Grave's disease.[89] This means that the test that is done for Grave's disease is compromised when one takes high dose biotin supplementation. This is important to consider, as someone who tests falsely positive for Grave's disease may be given anti-thyroid medication that could result in unrecognized hypothyroidism. In order to avoid this mistake, experts recommend stopping biotin supplementation two days before thyroid hormone testing.

Paleo Foods Rich in Biotin

Liver	Avocado
Eggs (if tolerated)	Raspberries
Salmon	Cauliflower

Folate (Vitamin B9)

Folate is an essential B vitamin that has been proven to protect against neural tube defects of an embryo during pregnancy. It also works with vitamin B12 to reduce homocysteine levels (a protein that has been associated with increased risk of cardiovascular disease as well as neurodegenerative diseases such as Alzheimer's). It is very important for the nervous system and is vital for reproductive health.

Folate is not to be confused with folic acid. Folate, otherwise referred to as vitamin B9, is naturally occurring in foods and can be metabolized by the intestine. Folic acid is the synthetic version that is used to fortify packaged foods. A study published in 2007 in the *Journal of the American Medical Association* showed that there was an increased risk of advanced cancer in a group of one thousand people supplementing with 1 milligram of folic acid per day.[91]

Folate deficiency.

Folate is very important for the development of a healthy neural tube as well as the heart and face of a growing fetus. Any woman of child-bearing age may recognize some of the symptoms listed below if a folate deficiency is present:

- Anemia
- Canker sores
- Diarrhea
- Fatigue
- Premature hair graying

Folate and hypothyroidism.

In general, people with hypothyroidism have higher homocysteine levels. Homocysteine is a protein found in the blood that, when high, is a risk factor for developing cardiovascular disease. Folate is one of the B vitamins that is responsible for lowering homocysteine levels in the blood. A 2012 study found that homocysteine levels were more effectively lowered by levothyroxine and folate in comparison to levothyroxine therapy alone. The authors recommended a combination therapy to lower homocysteine levels.[93]

Paleo Foods Rich in Folate

Organ meats	Avocado	Citrus fruits and juices
Spinach and green leafy vegetables in general	Asparagus	Broccoli
Poultry	Brussel Sprouts	Lettuce

How much folate is recommended?

The recommended daily intake for folate is 400 to 600 micrograms per day and is easily obtained from a diverse diet. If you do decide to supplement with folate, make sure to choose a whole food supplement in order to avoid the synthetic form.

Vitamin B12 (Cobalamine)

Vitamin B12 is essential for heart and mental health. Along with folate, it helps to reduce homocysteine levels in the blood and it boosts mood and energy and lowers one's risk for developing a neurodegenerative disease. It also helps with hair and nail health. Vitamin B12 helps the skin by reducing redness, dryness, inflammation and acne blemishes.

Vitamin B12 deficiency.

Vitamin B12 deficiency is very common worldwide and seems to be increasing. This is a common deficiency seen with Hashimoto's patients, as low levels of stomach acid associated with the disease decrease the absorption of B12 from food. Symptoms associated with the deficiency are as follows:

- Chronic fatigue
- Muscle aches and weakness
- Joint pain
- Shortness of breath
- Feeling dizzy
- Poor memory
- Inability to concentrate well
- Increased depression and anxiety
- Heart palpitations
- Bleeding gums and mouth sores
- Nausea, diarrhea, or cramping

If you have pernicious anemia, an autoimmune condition that attacks the cells that produce intrinsic factor (needed for vitamin B12 absorption) in your stomach, more serious symptoms like memory loss, confusion and long-term dementia can occur.

Vitamin B12 and hypothyroidism.

People with autoimmune thyroid disease are at higher risk of developing other autoimmune conditions, such as pernicious anemia, which decrease absorption of B12. Also, remember that low levels of stomach acid (also associated with this population) also decreases absorption of B12 from food. A recent review found that up to 55 percent of the people with Hashimoto's also have a vitamin B12 deficiency. The authors of the review recommended a B12 screening for all autoimmune thyroid patients as the prevalence of this deficiency is high in this population.[95]

Vitamin B12 is mainly found and better absorbed from animal foods. The amount of B12 that is actually absorbed depends on a person's digestive health. In the case of the hypothyroid population, I would recommend using a hydrochloric acid supplement with pepsin when eating vitamin B12-rich foods in order to ensure better absorption. Vegans definitely need to supplement with vitamin B12 in order to maintain optimal health.

Paleo foods rich in vitamin B12.

Beef and chicken liver	Mackerel	Trout
Salmon	Sardines	Turkey
Herring	Tuna	Lamb

Special note about vitamin B12 supplementation.

Many people with pernicious anemia are accustomed to getting intramuscular injections of vitamin B12 in order to increase its level in the blood. However, a recent review looking at the difference between oral supplementation of B12 and intramuscular injections found that supplementing with 1,000 micrograms of vitamin B12 is an adequate alternative to getting an injection.[96] Therefore, if you have a vitamin B12 deficiency, you should take 1,000 micrograms per day and test monthly to check its effect on your vitamin B12 status.

Vitamin B complex supplementation.

As all B vitamins work together to support a healthy metabolism, if you are thinking about a supplement, it's best to use a B-complex supplement. An example of the kind and quantities of B-vitamins that a supplement should have follow:

B Vitamin	Amount
Thiamine	5 mg
Riboflavin	10 mg
Niacin	35 mg
Pantothenic acid	45 mg
Vitamin B6	10 mg
Folate	450 mcg
Vitamin B12	133 mcg
Biotin	325 mcg

The above quantities vastly exceed the recommended daily intake of each B-vitamin. Upper limits of B-vitamins have only been established in studies for niacin at 35 milligrams, vitamin B6 at 100 milligrams and folate at 1,000 micrograms. However, when considering the vitamin deficiencies associated with thyroid disease as well as digestive and absorptive concerns, the above amounts should work well to optimize health.

Vitamins A, D, E and K as They Apply to Thyroid Health

Vitamin A

Vitamin A is a fat-soluble vitamin that helps to regulate immune responses; decreases inflammation in the body, as it is a powerful antioxidant; can prevent infections from developing; and is important for healthy skin, vision and neurological function.

Vitamin A deficiency.

According to Dr. Eric Osansky, an expert in treating hypothyroid and autoimmune thyroid disease, as far as the thyroid is concerned, thyroid hormone is needed to convert beta-carotene (a precursor of vitamin A) to vitamin A. Since there may not be enough thyroid hormone available for people with a hypothyroid condition, vitamin A is usually deficient in these individuals.

Signs of a vitamin A deficiency include the following:

- Poor eye health
- Premature skin damage
- Increased respiratory Infections
- Higher-risk pregnancy (night blindness during final trimester of pregnancy)

Vitamin A and the thyroid.

There is some research that shows supplementing with vitamin A can help to reduce TSH levels to normal. A randomized, double-blind controlled trial was conducted on eighty-four healthy women (fifty-four of whom were obese and twenty-eight of whom were of normal weight). Vitamin A supplementation caused a significant decrease in TSH in both groups. The authors of the study suggested that vitamin A supplementation might reduce the risk of subclinical hypothyroidism in premenopausal women.[100]

Another study suggested that supplementing with vitamin A could help to increase free T3 levels to normal when T3 is suppressed. This particular study aimed to look at how vitamin A and zinc deficiency affected thyroid abnormalities in people with hepatic and gastrointestinal disorders. The study concluded that there may be a causal relationship between deranged vitamin A metabolism and low T3 syndrome by interfering with either T4 entry into the tissues or the conversion of T4 to T3.[101]

Vitamin A metabolism is also affected by thyroid hormone status. Beta-carotene, a precursor to vitamin A, needs thyroid hormones to be converted.

Foods rich in vitamin A.

As taking too much supplemental vitamin A can be toxic, eating foods rich in vitamin A is your best bet for alleviating a vitamin A deficiency.

Paleo Foods Rich in Vitamin A

Cod liver oil	Egg yolks	Tuna fish
Organ meats	Kale	Apricots
Broccoli	Winter squash	Sweet red pepper

Vitamin A supplementation.

Supplementing with vitamin A can get confusing, as there are different forms of vitamin A. Pre-formed vitamin A comes in the form of retinol and retinyl ester and is found in foods like fish, meat and organ meats. Vitamin A can also come in the form of carotenoids like beta-carotene, alpha-carotene and beta-cryptoxanthin and is found in vegetables like sweet potatoes and carrots. This precursor of vitamin A is converted by the body into retinol.

The upper limit established by science that has not been known to show any adverse side effects is 10,000 IU or 3,000 mcg

RAE (retinol activity equivalents) per day. By 2019, all vitamin A supplements will be labelled in mcg RAE rather than IU's. If you do decide to take a supplement, you should know that 2 micrograms of beta-carotene is converted to 1 microgram of retinol. Therefore, if a supplement says that it contains 3,000 micrograms of beta-carotene, you are really getting 1,500 micrograms of vitamin A.

There is some debate as to whether vitamin A is, in fact, toxic if consumed in greater than 10,000 IU per day. Dr. Mary Enig, a nutritionist and researcher of lipids at the University of Maryland states that unless you are an arctic explorer and get huge amounts of vitamin A from eating polar bear liver, it is virtually impossible to overdose on vitamin A. You would either need to ingest 6 tablespoons of cod liver oil, a 250-gram serving of duck liver, 300 grams of beef liver or 309 egg yolks per day to get 100,000 IU from vitamin A. I doubt any of us has the problem of eating so much cod liver oil.

It is also important to note that if you get vitamin A from a synthetic beta-carotene source, you are getting just one of the fifty or sixty carotenes that are needed by the body to function. In fact, the biological activity of synthetic beta-carotene is much lower than that of natural carotene complexes and may put stress on the immune system. Therefore, always make sure to choose vitamin A supplements from a whole food source.

Vitamin D

Vitamin D seems to be the latest fad among health care professionals. However, the research is staggering as to how important vitamin D is for the immune system and how it can help prevent diseases like cancer, heart disease and diabetes. It is found in fish oils, eggs, fish such as salmon and sardines and cod liver oil or is made by the skin with exposure to the sun.

However, as mentioned previously, vitamin D metabolism and absorption can be impaired in people with hypothyroidism or autoimmune disease.

Vitamin D deficiency symptoms.

There are no clear-cut symptoms of vitamin D deficiency. However, the increase in vitamin D deficiency in recent years has been staggering. My children's pediatrician once told me that most of the children he sees are deficient in vitamin D, and we live in Cyprus, where there is sunshine most days of the year! Studies have found that Middle Eastern countries showed the same low levels of vitamin D.

According to Dr. Holick, an expert in vitamin D, over one billion people are either vitamin D deficient or insufficient.[106] In a recent study performed in India, 93 percent of healthy individuals were found to be vitamin D deficient. (This was defined as a serum 25 hydroxy vitamin D level of less than 20 ng/ml.) Considering the increase in vitamin D-related diseases, these numbers are really not surprising.[107]

Vitamin D and hypothyroidism.

Chris Kresser, a functional and integrative medicine practitioner and expert, says that any one of the following factors can contribute to impaired absorption of vitamin D:

- Since vitamin D is absorbed in the small intestine, a leaky and inflamed GI tract, which is extremely common in people with low thyroid function, reduces the absorption of vitamin D.

- High cortisol levels (caused by stress or medications like steroids) are associated with lower vitamin D levels. The synthesis of active vitamin D from sunlight depends on cholesterol. Stress hormones are also made from cholesterol. When the body is in an active stress response, most of the cholesterol is used to make cortisol and not enough is left over for vitamin D production.

- Obesity reduces the biological activity of vitamin D. Obese people have lower serum levels of vitamin D because it gets taken up by fat cells.

- Not eating enough fat or not digesting fat properly reduces absorption of vitamin D. Vitamin D is a fat-soluble vitamin, which means it requires fat to be absorbed. People on low-fat diets, and people with conditions that impair fat absorption (like irritable bowel syndrome, inflammatory bowel disease, gall bladder disease or liver disease) are more likely to have low levels of vitamin D.

- A variety of drugs reduce absorption or biologic activity of vitamin D. Unfortunately, these include drugs that are among the most popular and frequently prescribed, including antacids, replacement hormones, corticosteroids, anticoagulants and blood thinners.

- Aging reduces the conversion of sunlight to vitamin D

- Inflammation of any type reduces the utilization of vitamin D.

A 2013 study performed in Saudi Arabia found that vitamin D deficiency is significantly correlated with the degree and severity of hypothyroidism.[108]

There is evidence to show that vitamin D deficiency is even more common in people with Hashimoto's thyroiditis as vitamin D plays a pivotal role in immune balance.

Paleo Foods Rich in Vitamin D

Wild caught salmon	Sardines
Tuna	Free-range eggs
Mackerel	

Vitamin D supplementation.

There is not enough clinical evidence to recommend how high vitamin D levels should be in the blood in order to predict proper vitamin D absorption in the cells or to avoid vitamin D toxicity. It is important to know that vitamins A, D, and K2 work synergistically. Therefore, it may be possible to have higher levels of vitamin D in the blood if vitamin A and K2 are at normal levels. However, this is usually not the case in individuals with hypothyroidism. To find out how much vitamin D is appropriate for you, it is important to test your serum blood levels of 25 hydroxy vitamin D and work with your doctor to determine what level is appropriate for you.

However, having said this, the vitamin D council recommends that serum blood levels of vitamin D should be between 80 and100 ng/ml and that supplementing with 5,000 IU of vitamin D3 per day is recommended to achieve these levels. Only serum blood levels of 150 ng/ml are considered toxic levels of vitamin D.

Of course, sunshine is also a great way to get the ideal amount of vitamin D. (Please refer to chapter___ in order to get more specific directions as to how much sun exposure you need to optimize your vitamin D levels.)

Vitamin E

Vitamin E is a powerful antioxidant that helps to protect against cancer and cardiovascular disease. It is made up of four tocopherols and four tocotrienols.

Vitamin E deficiency symptoms.

Vitamin E deficiencies are rare and typically occur with inflammatory bowel disease such as Crohn's disease, liver disease or pancreatic insufficiency. Symptoms can include loss of muscle coordination and impaired vision and speech.

Paleo Foods Rich in Vitamin E

Avocado	Olive oil	Almonds
Butternut squash	Spinach	Sunflower seeds
Broccoli	Kiwi	Hazelnuts

Vitamin E and thyroid health.

Vitamin E, along with other synergistic minerals such as selenium, helps to convert T4 to T3. Therefore, if one has vitamin E insufficiency, it becomes harder for this transition to take place.

One study showed that synthroid medication with vitamin E helped with cognitive function and decreasing oxidative stress (as compared to the medication by itself).

Vitamin E supplementation.

If you decide to supplement with vitamin E, make sure to take a whole food supplement with the entire vitamin E complex. Many available vitamin E supplements include alpha-tocopherol only, which alone does not produce any health benefits.

A study done to determine the effects of vitamin E on liver disease found that giving 400 IU of mixed tocotrienols significantly improved outcomes and increased the amount of vitamin E found in human tissues. The average duration of the study was for twenty weeks, with no noted adverse effects.[112]

The Recommended Daily Allowance for vitamin E is 22.4 IU per day. The tolerable upper intake is 1,500 IU per day. It is very important to talk to your doctor about vitamin E supplementation before you begin, as there have been some studies that link high doses (300 to 800 IU) of vitamin E supplementation with adverse effects in people with heart disease or diabetes.

Vitamin K

Vitamin K comes in two forms, vitamin K1, which is found mainly in plant-based foods, and vitamin K2 which comes from animal-based foods. Vitamin K1 is important for proper blood clotting while vitamin K2 plays an important role in the absorption of calcium and therefore the prevention of osteoporosis.

Vitamin K2 can be produced in the intestine; however, if there is decreased intestinal functioning (as is common with thyroid disease) from issues like SIBO or IBD, vitamin K2 deficiency can occur. Therefore, healing the gut would play a large part in alleviating a vitamin K2 deficiency and therefore in the prevention of osteoporosis. Vitamin K2 supplementation can definitely be warranted in thyroid disease.

Vitamin K deficiency.

Vitamin K deficiency can lead to heart disease, weakened bones, tooth decay, and cancer. As previously mentioned, it is imperative to heal the gut so that sufficient amounts of vitamin K are absorbed into the blood via the intestine.

Vitamin K and thyroid health.

What role does the thyroid play in vitamin K metabolism? It plays a part in vitamin K1 metabolism which has to do with clotting. Therefore, people who have hypothyroidism have a decrease in blood clotting and an increased risk of bleeding.

Paleo Foods that Contain Vitamin K:

Vitamin K2 can be produced in the intestine; however, if there is decreased intestinal functioning (as is common with thyroid disease) from issues like SIBO or IBD, vitamin K2 deficiency can occur. Therefore, healing the gut would play a large part in alleviating a vitamin K2 deficiency and therefore in the prevention of osteoporosis. Vitamin K2 supplementation can definitely be warranted in thyroid disease.

Vitamin K deficiency.

Vitamin K deficiency can lead to heart disease, weakened bones, tooth decay, and cancer. As previously mentioned, it is imperative to heal the gut so that sufficient amounts of vitamin K are absorbed into the blood via the intestine.

Vitamin K and thyroid health.

What role does the thyroid play in vitamin K metabolism? It plays a part in vitamin K1 metabolism which has to do with clotting. Therefore, people who have hypothyroidism have a decrease in blood clotting and an increased risk of bleeding.

Paleo Foods that Contain Vitamin K:

Vitamin K2 can be produced in the intestine; however, if there is decreased intestinal functioning (as is common with thyroid disease) from issues like SIBO or IBD, vitamin K2 deficiency can occur. Therefore, healing the gut would play a large part in alleviating a vitamin K2 deficiency and therefore in the prevention of osteoporosis. Vitamin K2 supplementation can definitely be warranted in thyroid disease.

Vitamin K deficiency.

Vitamin K deficiency can lead to heart disease, weakened bones, tooth decay, and cancer. As previously mentioned, it is imperative to heal the gut so that sufficient amounts of vitamin K are absorbed into the blood via the intestine.

Vitamin K and thyroid health.

What role does the thyroid play in vitamin K metabolism? It plays a part in vitamin K1 metabolism which has to do with clotting. Therefore, people who have hypothyroidism have a decrease in blood clotting and an increased risk of bleeding.

Vitamin K2 can be produced in the intestine; however, if there is decreased intestinal functioning (as is common with thyroid disease) from issues like SIBO or IBD, vitamin K2 deficiency can occur. Therefore, healing the gut would play a large part in alleviating a vitamin K2 deficiency and therefore in the prevention of osteoporosis. Vitamin K2 supplementation can definitely be warranted in thyroid disease.

Vitamin K deficiency.

Vitamin K deficiency can lead to heart disease, weakened bones, tooth decay, and cancer. As previously mentioned, it is imperative to heal the gut so that sufficient amounts of vitamin K are absorbed into the blood via the intestine.

Vitamin K and thyroid health.

What role does the thyroid play in vitamin K metabolism? It

plays a part in vitamin K1 metabolism which has to do with clotting. Therefore, people who have hypothyroidism have a decrease in blood clotting and an increased risk of bleeding.

Paleo Foods that Contain Vitamin K:

Dandelion greens	Brussel sprouts	Broccoli
Mustard greens	Spinach	Asparagus
Swiss chard	Kale	Cucumbers

Vitamin K supplementation

The Recommended Daily Allowance for vitamin K for adults is 90 micrograms per day. Taking more than this could interfere with the proper absorption of vitamins A and E, and therefore getting more than the RDA for vitamin K is unnecessary. Please note that you should not take vitamin K supplements or even decrease the amount of vitamin K-containing foods you eat if you are on blood-thinning drugs, have experienced a stroke or cardiac arrest, or are prone to blood clotting. As always, speak with your doctor before starting a vitamin K supplement.

Tyrosine

Tyrosine is a non essential amino acid that can be obtained from food or produced by the body on its own. Remember from chapter one that tyrosine is needed to form thyroid hormones. Therefore, supplementation with tyrosine could play a role in natural thyroid therapy.

CHAPTER 6

SEVEN-STEP GUIDE TO EATING FOR A HEALTHY THYROID

Ok, so now you have read about how nutrition can affect the thyroid. Now what? When I was at my lowest with my hypothyroid condition, I would pray that even a small beacon of light would come to me so that I could start to feel better. That moment came when I discovered that changing my diet made me feel better in a matter of days.

The truth is that I could sit here and tell you how easy it is to change your diet. However, realistically, it is one of the hardest things you will ever do. We are creatures of habit and we are easily enticed, so it takes a lot of determination to go against what we are used to doing.

However, we are also capable of completely revamping our lifestyles to ultimately be "reborn." The road is not easy, but it is so worth it.

I, along with other thyroid experts, have basically told you to get rid of grains and dairy products from your diet. Most of you reading this are probably thinking, "Man, these foods are what my diet is predominantly made up of. How will I live without these foods?!" The answer is, one step at a time.

Here is a seven-step guide I have created to get you on the path to eating for a healthy thyroid. You should know that you could at any point find yourself backtracking and starting over from step 1. However, this guide was devised so that you can get back on track, even if you falter.

Step 1:

Have a Going-Away Party

For one full week, make dishes, snacks and desserts that you think you will miss. Just go for the works. Make pizza for dinner on one night, chocolate-chip cookies for dessert the following night and a plate of pasta the next. This may sound a bit unorthodox, but while eating these foods, at the same time say goodbye and make your peace with the fact that you are trading these foods in for your health.

Step 2:

What Foods Are in Your Pantry?

Take a few days to take stock of what foods you typically fill your house with and try to replace common foods with foods that will boost thyroid health. Below are some of my recommendations:

Instead of....	Try this....
Conventional bread	Bread made from almond butter and coconut flour
Conventional chocolates	Homemade chocolate bars
Crackers and biscuits	Gluten-free crackers and biscuits (to be used sparingly)
Flour	Coconut or almond flour
Breakfast cereals and bars	Free- range eggs and homemade bars made from dates and nuts
Conventional meat, poultry, fish and seafood	Organic and grass-fed meat and poultry and wild-caught fish and seafood
Anything in a box with more than four ingredients	Anything in a box with fewer than four ingredients (in other words, get rid of all processed foods).

Step 3:

Create a Budget and Do Some Research

You always want to make sure that the way you eat is feasible in terms of your lifestyle as well as your wallet. Establish a comfortable amount you would like to spend on food and then do some research to organize how you will eat throughout the week. This particular step will need to be repeated weekly so that you can plan your weekly shopping.

Research includes looking for recipes that are gluten- and dairy-free. Here's a tip: any dish made from vegetables and fresh meat, poultry and fish are naturally gluten-free. Not much imagination needed here. Research also includes taking into consideration how much time and preparation you will allot for meal preparation and planning. For many, this will be similar each week, but for others, it can vary greatly. The point here is to dedicate some time each week to researching, shopping for and preparing your meals and snacks so that you will be ready during your busy schedule throughout the week.

Step 4:

Be Prepared for Eating Out and Special Occasions

This is the step that most of my clients (including myself in the past) struggle with. Again, a little research and preparation here can go a long way. Take the time to find restaurants and cafes in your area that offer a gluten-free menu as well as restaurants that are willing to accommodate your special nutrition needs. (This way, when a friend suggests you eat out, you can be prepared with a list of restaurants that you prefer.)

When it comes to special occasions and holidays, find out what foods will be available before you go. This way, if there will be no desserts you can have, you can volunteer to bring your own dessert that will be made according to your nutritional needs (and no one has to know it's gluten- or dairy-free!)

Step 5:

Get Moving

Exercise is always a great way to gain energy and to feel better. However, as we have spoken about in this book, you need to find an exercise that is calming as well health-enhancing. Incorporating low- to moderate-intensity activities such as walking, weight training, pilates or yoga into your routine will help you to increase your physical activity, help you to manage stress and encourage you to continue your newfound eating habits.

Step 6:

Reach Out for Help

Changing your lifestyle is challenging and no man is an island. We all need support and encouragement when things get tough. Find online forums of other hypothyroid patients making similar changes from whom to ask questions and get ideas. Involve family members and friends in your new journey to get their feedback as well as their support. Seek the advice of a trusted health care professional to get the answers you need when you want them. Support is what gets most of us through the day, week, month, year and decades. Don't be afraid to ask. Help is everywhere.

Step 7:

Don't Be So Hard on Yourself

Let's face it. We are all human and are bound to go back to the way we were used to eating at one point or another. Many thyroid experts will tell you that you *have* to remain gluten- and dairy-free in order to see results. Although this may be true, in my experience, most people falter for whatever reason. This step is for you to realize that even though you may have slipped up, you need to forgive yourself and just keep moving in the right direction. Eventually, you will get to a point where you will never eat gluten or dairy again.

Putting It All Together

Taking matters of health that you can control, like your diet, into your own hands can seem daunting and quite overwhelming. However, you already took the first step by reading this book. Now all you have to do is to take the next steps. In the following pages, I briefly describe what to do to start feeling better (and less tired) within a matter of weeks.

Begin With An Elimination Diet

The following foods are foods that you should eliminate for at least one month. You may experience some symptoms of detoxification within the first few days of elimination, like headaches, lightheadedness, dizziness, or muscular aches and pains. But don't worry, this is just your body's way of getting rid of deleterious, inflammation-causing toxins. This process is quite similar to weaning off of drugs like cocaine (not that I am suggesting anyone should take drugs), your body gets rid of the toxic drug by sweating and aching. However, once the beginning of getting rid of inflammation-causing foods is finished, you really start to see the value of eating a clean diet. The best way I can describe what you will feel is that within days, you will have more clarity and feel more energy. You will literally feel your body come back to life.

Here are the foods you need to eliminate:

1. **Gluten-containing foods** predominantly from wheat, rye and barley (refer to chapter 5 for a more comprehensive list).

2. **All dairy.**

3. **Soy.** This includes miso, tempeh, edamame, soy milk and any processed foods with soy additives like soy lecithin.

4. **Sugar.** Avoid any processed baked goods, sweets, and processed foods in general. Sugar can be hidden in foods like ketchup, tomato sauce, and gluten-free bread. The only form of sugar you should get is from fruit. I recommend two to three fruits per day.

5. **Common genetically modified foods.** This includes wheat and soy, which are already excluded, but another food to look out for is corn. Corn is another crop that is predominantly genetically modified, so steer clear from corn and its products in processed foods. If you do choose to eat corn, make sure it's organic.

6. **Pesticides and insecticides.** It is *very* important to choose organic fruits and vegetables as the chemicals sprayed on conventionally-grown fruits and vegetables are endocrine disruptors and can hinder thyroid function. Make sure to

get organically-raised meat and poultry and choose wild-caught fish and seafood.

7. **Alcohol.** Although you may think that the occasional glass of wine or beer may not be a big deal, it *is* when you are trying to heal. So, for the month, try to stay away from any alcoholic beverages.

8. **Nuts and Seeds.** These are forbidden on an autoimmune Paleo protocol because they can exacerbate conditions associated with an inflamed intestinal tract and can act as a trigger to Hashimoto's thyroiditis.

9. **Nightshade Vegetables.** Like nuts and seeds, nightshade vegetables should be eliminated on an autoimmune Paleo protocol because they can trigger symptoms associated with autoimmunity. Please refer to chapter 5 for a more extensive list of nightshade fruits and vegetables.

10. **Eggs.** The yolks of the eggs may be added back after the month is over.

Foods you can include when doing your elimination diet:

1. **Organic and grass-fed meat and poultry** (anything is ok as long as it is organically sourced, even bacon!) An interesting point here is that grass-fed meat is typically organic, however, meat labeled as organic is not necessarily grass-fed. This could create a problem because if an animal is given feed from grains, this increases the omega 6 to omega 3 ratio, which causes more inflammation. Exclusively pasture-raised meat is a good source of omega 3 fatty acids.

2. **Offal.** These include organ meats like the liver, the brain, the bones, the fat, and even head meat. Each part of the animal offers different nutrients needed to heal.

3. **Wild-caught fish and seafood.** Buying farm-raised fish is dangerous because they are given genetically-modified feed. Buying wild-caught fish and seafood definitely reduces your exposure to chemicals that can hurt your thyroid.

4. **Fruits and vegetables.** The sky is the limit here. Choose a variety of fruits and vegetables daily in order to enhance the nutrient density you are getting. Do not be afraid of goitrogenic vegetables like broccoli or cauliflower because, as discussed in chapter 5, these foods do not hinder thyroid activity when cooked and have nutrients that help the body to detoxify.

269

5. **Coconut oil and Olive oil.** These are really the only two oils you need in order to heal Make sure to add these two oils to salads, vegetables, smoothies, and any recipe that calls for a little bit of oil.

6. **Plenty of filtered water.** It is important to get at least 2 liters of *clean* water per day in order to help your body clean out toxins and remain well hydrated. Make sure to drink water in between meals and not during meals. Water intake while eating can dilute the acid in the stomach (needed to sufficiently break your food down).

Here is a list of foods that you can use to start planning some recipes:

Fish	Seafood
• Anchovy, arctic char, atlantic croaker • Barcheek goby, bass, bonito, bream, brill, brisling • Carp, catfish, cod, conger, common dab, crappie, croaker • Drum, eel, fera, filefish, gar, haddock, hake halibut, herring • John Dory, king mackerel • Lamprey, ling, loach • Marlin, mackerel, mahi-mahi, milkfish, minnow, monkfish, mullet • Pandora, perch, plaice, Pollock • Sailfish, salmon, sardine, shad, shark	• Abalone • Clams • Cockles • Conch • Crab • Crawfish • Cuttlefish • Limpets • Lobster • Mussels • Octopus • Oysters • Scallops • Shrimp • Snails • Squid • Periwinkles • Whelks • Anemone • Jellyfish

• Sheepshead, silverside, smelt, snakehead, snapper, sole, swordfish • Tarpin, tilapia, tilefish, trout, tub gurnaurd, tuna, turbot, walleye, whiting	• Sea cucumber • Sea squirt • Sea urchin • Starfish

Meat and Poultry	Offal
• Beef (veal), pork, and lamb • Antelope, bear, beaver, buffalo, boar • Camel, caribou, deer • Elk, goat, hare, kangaroo, moose • Rabbit • Chicken, dove, duck • Emu, goose, grouse • Pigeon, pheasant, quail • Turkey	• Bone marrow, bones to make bone broth • Heart, kidneys, liver, tripe (stomach), melt (spleen), rinds (skin) • Brains • Chitterlings and intestines • Head meat • Fats like lard • Tail and tongue

Vegetables	
• Arugula	• Artichoke
• Broccoli rabe	• Asparagus
• Cabbage	• Broccoli
• Celery	• Caper
• Collard greens	• Cauliflower
• Cress	• Fennel
• Dandelion greens	• Rhubarb
• Kohlrabi greens	• Chive
• :ettuce	• Garlic
• Mustard greens	• Onion
• Radicchio	• Scallion
• Sea kale	• Arrowroot
• Plantain	• Beet
• Pumpkin	• Carrot
• Squash	• Ginger
• Winter melon	• Parsnip
	• Radish
	• Avocad
	• Cucumber
	• Okra
	• Zucchini

Fruits	
• Acai	• Apple
• Blackberry	• Apricot
• Blueberry	• Cherry
• Cranberry	• Loquat
• Elderberry	• Peach
• Grape	• Pear
• Lingonberry	• Plum
• Raspberry	• Clementine
• Sea buckthorn	• Grapefruit
• Strawberry	• Lemon
• Cantaloupe	• Lime
• Melon pear	• Kumquat
• Watermelon	• Mango
• Passion fruit	• Papaya
• Guava	• Kiwi

These lists were adapted from Dr. Sarah Ballantyne's book, The Paleo Approach. For a more extensive list of these foods, please refer to pages 201 to 205 of her book.

The best advice I can give at this point is to not be afraid to try new things even if you may think they are disgusting or not appetizing. Remember, the more variety that you include, the more nutrients you are providing to your body to help it to heal. Make sure to eat greens at every meal as green leafy vegetables boost the antioxidant capacity of the diet and contain phytonutrients that prevent red meat from producing toxic products in the gut. You always want to mix some meat, poultry or seafood with a variety of vegetables (especially from greens).

Do you need some recipe ideas in order to create tasty recipes with the above foods? Check out these websites:

www.grazedandenthused.com

www.thepaleomom.com

www.primalpalate.com

www.aiplifestyle.com

All of these websites were created by pioneers in healing autoimmune disorders with food. You can choose from many delicious recipes, including breakfast and desserts.

Recommended Supplements

Many nutritionists argue that all you need to heal is a full and diverse diet. Although this is the ideal scenario, realistically, most people need a boost in nutrients in order to heal. The following are my recommendations for when and how much of specific supplements you should take to help heal Hashimoto's thyroiditis:

<u>On an empty stomach:</u>

Thyroxine (This quantity is determined by your doctor)

Selenium 200 mcg

Vitamin E 400 IU

Probiotics (make sure to start with a count of about 5 billion and increase by 5 billion every three days. Work your way up to 50 billion per day.) It is important to note that you will most likely need a professional grade of probiotics to heal. If you do not have access to this, the next best thing is to order a starter kit of probiotics and to ferment vegetables or create coconut water kefir with it. This boosts the number of naturally occurring probiotics to the trillions, which happens to be the ideal amount needed to heal.

Any adrenal adaptogens you may need. (Remember that taking licorice in the morning and taking ashwaganda and holy basil leaf at night is preferable. The quantity should be determined by you and your functional medicine practitioner).

With Breakfast:

HCl supplement with digestive enzymes (refer to chapter 1 to understand dosage)

Glutamine supplement OR collagen supplement. Glutamine is better in powder form. Take about 5 grams. Collagen powders should be grass-fed. You can add them to your meals or in a smoothie.

With Lunch:

HCl supplement with enzymes

B-complex vitamin

Zinc 25 to 50 mg

Vitamin D3 5,000 IU

Collagen powder

Fish oil from small fish like anchovies (Some fish oils are already mixed with olive leaf extract. If they are not, include olive oil in your meal to protect against the oxidization of the fish oils).

<u>With Dinner:</u>

HCl supplement with enzymes

Collagen powder

<u>Before bedtime:</u>

Magnesium 300mg – 500mg

What to Do After the One Month Elimination Diet

I often recommend to clients to follow the autoimmune diet protocol for at least three months. Therefore, if you have gotten used to eating in this way after one month, I would continue. If you would like to test your tolerance to certain foods, now is the time when you can add back certain foods like nuts, seeds, and egg yolks. In order to add back these foods, add them one at a time and allow a few days to pass in between. For example, try almonds on one day and then egg yolks after three days. Keep a journal to write down any noticed reactions. If you notice that some symptoms continue, for example, you eat almonds and you get bloated, continue to exclude them from your diet.

After one to three months, you can also start experimenting with gluten-free grains like quinoa, buckwheat, millet, and oats.

But, note that these should be used sparingly as they too can trigger autoimmune responses in sensitive individuals. At this stage, you can also try to re-introduce beans, pulses, and lentils as well. These foods should be eaten on occasion if tolerated in order to allow the intestinal tract to heal.

The duration of the autoimmune protocol usually depends on the severity of one's symptoms and issues. I have had clients see improvements in as little as one month and clients that needed one to two years to be able to add back foods and tolerate them. Therefore, make sure that you keep track of what you are eating and how you react to certain foods, in order to be able to add back more foods later.

These are the nutrition basics for getting you started on the road to recovery. I know it is challenging, however, once you start to regain your health and your energy, you will never want to go back to how you used to eat.

Final Thoughts

When people have hypothyroidism, they may feel like their lives are over. This is so because they gain weight, they feel depressed, they lose hair, and they are tired all the time. They yearn to feel alive and full of energy like they once did. I know because I, too, was one of them.

Make the decision to not be a hypothyroid victim and take

control of your health and well-being. Overcome not feeling well all the time and make the commitment to change your diet and your lifestyle. Join the many people, including myself, who have transformed their lives for the better. Don't settle for "good enough" as a standard of living. Rise above and you will conquer. You and only you have the power to do this.

REFERENCES

Chapter 1: Thyroid Disease Basics

1. Mark P. J. Vanderpump. "The epidemiology of thyroid disease." BR MED BULL 99, no. 1 (2011): 39-51.

2. Vanderpump MPJ. Braverman LE, Utiger RD. "The epidemiology of thyroid diseases." *Werner and Ingbar's The Thyroid: A Fundamental and Clinical Text*, 2005 9th edition, Philadelphia, JB Lippincott-Raven (pg. 298-496)

3. Biondi, Bernadette, and David S. Cooper. "The clinical significance of subclinical thyroid dysfunction." *Endocrine reviews* 29, no. 1 (2008): 76-131.

4. Tunbridge, W. M. G., D. C. Evered, R. Hall, D. Appleton, M. Brewis, F. Clark, J. Grimley Evans, E. Young, T. Bird, and P. A. Smith. "The spectrum of thyroid disease in a community: the Whickham survey." *Clinical endocrinology* 7, no. 6 (1977): 481-493.

5. Canaris, Gay J., Neil R. Manowitz, Gilbert Mayor, and E. Chester Ridgway. "The Colorado thyroid disease prevalence study." *Archives of internal medicine* 160, no. 4 (2000): 526-534.

6. Kresser, Chris. "Thyroid Disorders." http://my.chriskresser.com/wp-content/uploads/membership-files/ebooks/Thyroid%20Disorders.pdf?_ga=1.24399865.2 94555743.1467052812 (Accessed September 8, 2016).

7. Wentz, Isabella. "The Common Root Cause of Hashimoto's Hives and IBS." http://thyroidpharmacist.com/articles/the-common-root-cause-of-hashimotos-hives-and-ibs (Accessed May 4, 2016).

8. Haskell, ND. Hope for Hasimoto's, Advancing Medical Care Inc. 2011

Chapter 2: The Gut Connection

1. World's Healthies Foods. "How Does Digestion work and how can I improve mine?" http://www.whfoods.com/genpage.php?tname=faq&dbid=16 (Accessed January 7, 2016).

2. Course Notes. *Symptomatology.* (2011). The Institute of Holistic Nutrition.

3. Myhill (2014), Hypochlorhydria – lack of stomach acid – can cause lots of problems http://drmyhill.co.uk/wiki/hypochlorhydria_-_lack_of_stomach_acid_-_can_cause_lots_of_problems [Accessed January 8th, 2016]

4. Centanni, Marco, Massimo Marignani, Lucilla Gargano, Vito D. Corleto, Alessandro Casini, Gianfranco Delle Fave, Mario Andreoli, and Bruno Annibale. "Atrophic body gastritis in patients with autoimmune thyroid

disease: an underdiagnosed association." *Archives of internal medicine* 159, no. 15 (1999): 1726-1730.

5. Bohm, Matthew, Robert M. Siwiec, and John M. Wo. "Diagnosis and management of small intestinal bacterial overgrowth." *Nutrition in Clinical Practice* (2013): 0884533613485882.

6. Al-Kaade, S. "Etiology of Exocrine Pancreatic Insufficiency." http://emedicine.medscape.com/article/2121028-overview#aw2aab6b2b4 (Accessed January 8, 2016).

7. Kresser, Chris. "Pioneering Researcher Alessio Fasano M.D. on Gluten, Autoimmunity and Leaky Gut." http://chriskresser.com/pioneering-researcher-alessio-fasano-m-d-on-gluten-autoimmunity-leaky-gut (Accessed January 11, 2016).

8. Galland L. "Leaky gut syndromes: Breaking the vicious cycle." http://www.mdheal.org/leakygut.htm (Accessed January 11, 2016).

9. Wentz, I, Nowosadzka, M, *Hashimoto's Thyroiditis, Lifestyle Interventions for Finding and Treating the Root Cause.* [Wentz, LLC, 2013], 73-75.

10. Anderson, James M., and Christina M. Van Itallie. "Physiology and function of the tight junction." *Cold Spring Harbor perspectives in biology* 1, no. 2 (2009): a002584.

11. Fasano, Alessio. "Leaky gut and autoimmune diseases." *Clinical reviews in allergy & immunology* 42, no. 1 (2012): 71-78.

12. Lloyd-Price, Jason, Galeb Abu-Ali, and Curtis Huttenhower. "The healthy human microbiome." *Genome medicine* 8, no. 1 (2016): 51.

13. Yu, Jingcheng, and Ronald J. Koenig. "Regulation of hepatocyte thyroxine 5'-deiodinase by T3 and nuclear receptor coactivators as a model of the sick euthyroid syndrome." *Journal of Biological Chemistry* 275, no. 49 (2000): 38296-38301.

14. Byrne, C. S., E. S. Chambers, D. J. Morrison, and G. Frost. "The role of short chain fatty acids in appetite regulation and energy homeostasis." *International journal of obesity* 39, no. 9 (2015): 1331-1338.

15. Frost, Gary, Michelle L. Sleeth, Meliz Sahuri-Arisoylu, Blanca Lizarbe, Sebastian Cerdan, Leigh Brody, Jelena Anastasovska et al. "The short-chain fatty acid acetate reduces appetite via a central homeostatic mechanism." *Nature communications* 5 (2014).

16. Duncan, Sylvia H., Petra Louis, John M. Thomson, and Harry J. Flint. "The role of pH in determining the species composition of the human colonic microbiota." *Environmental microbiology* 11, no. 8 (2009): 2112-2122.

17. Malo, Madhu S., Wenying Zhang, Fuad Alkhoury, Premraj Pushpakaran, Mario A. Abedrapo, Moushumi Mozumder, Elizabeth Fleming, Aleem Siddique, Joseph W. Henderson, and Richard A. Hodin. "Thyroid hormone positively regulates the enterocyte differentiation marker intestinal alkaline phosphatase gene via an atypical response element." *Molecular Endocrinology* 18, no. 8 (2004): 1941-1962.

18. Veiga, Patrick, Carey Ann Gallini, Chloé Beal, Monia Michaud, Mary L. Delaney, Andrea DuBois, Artem Khlebnikov et al. "Bifidobacterium animalis subsp. lactis fermented milk product reduces inflammation by altering a niche for colitogenic microbes." *Proceedings of the National Academy of Sciences* 107, no. 42 (2010): 18132-18137.

19. Derrien, Muriel, and Johan ET van Hylckama Vlieg. "Fate, activity, and impact of ingested bacteria within the human gut microbiota." *Trends in microbiology* 23, no. 6 (2015): 354-366.

20. Varian, B. J., T. Poutahidis, T. Levkovich, Y. M. Ibrahim, J. R. Lakritz, A. Chatzigiagkos, A. Scherer-Hoock, E. J. Alm, and S. E. Erdman. "Beneficial bacteria stimulate youthful thyroid gland activity." *Journal of Obesity & Weight Loss Therapy* 4, no. 2 (2014).

21. Manolakis, C.S. et al. "Small Intestinal Bacterial Overgrowth" In *GI/Liver Secrets Plus*, p 334. Fifth Edition. New Dehli, Saunders, Elsevier, 2015.

22. Vojdani, A., P. Rahimian, H. Kalhor, and E. Mordechai. "Immunological cross reactivity between Candida albicans and human tissue." *Journal of clinical & laboratory immunology* 48, no. 1 (1995): 1-15.

23. Axe, Josh. "9 Candida Symptoms and 3 Steps to Treat Them." http://draxe.com/candida-symptoms/ (Accessed February 2, 2016).

24. Fukushima, Chizu, Hiroto Matsuse, Shinya Tomari, Yasushi Obase, Yoshitsugu Miyazaki, Terufumi Shimoda, and Shigeru Kohno. "Oral candidiasis associated with inhaled corticosteroid use: comparison of fluticasone and beclomethasone." *Annals of Allergy, Asthma & Immunology* 90, no. 6 (2003): 646-651.

25. DiNubile, Mark J., Darcy Hille, Carole A. Sable, and Nicholas A. Kartsonis. "Invasive candidiasis in cancer patients: observations from a randomized clinical trial." *Journal of Infection* 50, no. 5 (2005): 443-449.

26. Fichtenbaum, Carl J. and Aberg, "Judith A. Candidiasis and HIV." http://hivinsite.ucsf.edu/InSite%3Fpage%3Dkb-00%26doc%3Dkb-05-02-03 (Accessed February 2, 2016).

27. Shmuely, Haim, Noam Domniz, and Jacob Yahav. "Non-pharmacological treatment of Helicobacter pylori." *World journal of gastrointestinal pharmacology and therapeutics* 7, no. 2 (2016): 171.

28. Fahey, Jed W., Katherine K. Stephenson, and Alison J. Wallace. "Dietary amelioration of Helicobacter infection." *Nutrition Research* 35, no. 6 (2015): 461-473.

29. Thung, I., H. Aramin, V. Vavinskaya, S. Gupta, J. Y. Park, S. E. Crowe, and M. A. Valasek. "Review article: the global emergence of Helicobacter pylori antibiotic resistance." *Alimentary pharmacology & therapeutics* 43, no. 4 (2016): 514-533.

30. de Luis, Daniel A., César Varela, H. de La Calle, Rafael Cantón, Carlos Martin de Argila, Antonio L. San Roman, and Daniel Boixeda. "Helicobacter pylori infection is markedly increased in patients with autoimmune atrophic thyroiditis." *Journal of clinical gastroenterology* 26, no. 4 (1998): 259-263.

31. Xiao, Shu Dong, and Tong Shi. "Is cranberry juice effective in the treatment and prevention of Helicobacter pylori infection of mice?." *Chinese Journal of Digestive Diseases* 4, no. 3 (2003): 136-139.

32. Chatterjee, Archana, Taharat Yasmin, Debasis Bagchi, and Sidney J. Stohs. "Inhibition of Helicobacter pylori in vitro by various berry extracts, with enhanced susceptibility to

clarithromycin." *Molecular and cellular biochemistry* 265, no. 1 (2004): 19-26.

33. Shmuely, Haim, Ora Burger, Itzhak Neeman, Jacob Yahav, Zmira Samra, Yaron Niv, Nathan Sharon et al. "Susceptibility of Helicobacter pylori isolates to the antiadhesion activity of a high-molecular-weight constituent of cranberry." *Diagnostic microbiology and infectious disease* 50, no. 4 (2004): 231-235.

34. Kundu, Parag, Ronita De, Ipsita Pal, Asish K. Mukhopadhyay, Dhira Rani Saha, and Snehasikta Swarnakar. "Curcumin alleviates matrix metalloproteinase-3 and-9 activities during eradication of Helicobacter pylori infection in cultured cells and mice." *PloS one* 6, no. 1 (2011): e16306.

35. Prucksunand Chaweewan, Bunjob Indrasukhsri, Manit Leethochawalit, and Korpong Hungspreugs. "Phase II clinical trial on effect of the long turmeric (Curcuma longa Linn) on healing of peptic ulcer." (2001).

36. Mahady, Gail B., Susan L. Pendland Gina S. Yun, Zhi-Zhen Lu, and Adina Stoia. "Ginger (Zingiber officinale Roscoe) and the gingerols inhibit the growth of Cag A+ strains of Helicobacter pylori." *Anticancer research* 23 (2003): 3699.

37. Gaus, Kristen, Yue Huang, Dawn A. Israel, Susan L. Pendland Bolanle A. Adeniyi, and Gail B. Mahady.

"Standardized ginger (Zingiber officinale) extract reduces bacterial load and suppresses acute and chronic inflammation in Mongolian gerbils infected with cagA+ Helicobacter pylori." *Pharmaceutical biology* 47, no. 1 (2009): 92-98.

38. Al-Said, Mansoor S., A. M. Ageel, N. S. Parmar, and M. Tariq. "Evaluation of mastic, a crude drug obtained from Pistacia lentiscus for gastric and duodenal anti-ulcer activity." *Journal of ethnopharmacology* 15, no. 3 (1986): 271-278.

39. Al-Habbal, Mohammad Jamil, Zakaria Al-Habbal, and Farhad Umer Huwez. "A Double-Blind Controlled Clinical Trial of Mastic and Placebo in the Treatment of Duodenal Ulcer." *Clinical and experimental pharmacology and physiology* 11, no. 5 (1984): 541-544.

40. Huwez, Farhad U., Debbie Thirlwell, Alan Cockayne, and Dlawer AA Ala'Aldeen. "Mastic gum kills Helicobacter pylori." *New England Journal of Medicine* 339, no. 26 (1998): 1946-1946.

41. Choli-Papadopoulou, Theodora, Filippos Kottakis, Georgios Papadopoulos, and Stefanos Pendas. "Helicobacter pylori neutrophil activating protein as target for new drugs against H. pylori inflammation." *World J Gastroenterol* 17, no. 21 (2011): 2585-2591.

42. Dabos, K. J., E. Sfika, L. J. Vlatta, and G. Giannikopoulos. "The effect of mastic gum on

Helicobacter pylori: a randomized pilot study." *Phytomedicine* 17, no. 3 (2010): 296-299.

43. Marone, P., L. Bono, E. Leone, S. Bona, E. Carretto, and L. Perversi. "Bactericidal activity of Pistacia lentiscus mastic gum against Helicobacter pylori." *Journal of Chemotherapy* 13, no. 6 (2001): 611-614.

44. Fahey, Jed W., Xavier Haristoy, Patrick M. Dolan, Thomas W. Kensler, Isabelle Scholtus, Katherine K. Stephenson, Paul Talalay, and Alain Lozniewski. "Sulforaphane inhibits extracellular, intracellular, and antibiotic-resistant strains of Helicobacter pylori and prevents benzo [a] pyrene-induced stomach tumors." *Proceedings of the National Academy of Sciences* 99, no. 11 (2002): 7610-7615.

45. Yanaka, A., M. Tauchi, and M. Yamamoto. "Effects of sulforaphane-rich broccoli sprouts on H. pylori-infected gastric mucosa." *Nihon rinsho. Japanese journal of clinical medicine* 63 (2005): 582.

46. Bahadoran, Zahra, Parvin Mirmiran, Maryam Zarif Yeganeh, Farhad Hosseinpanah, Homayoun Zojaji, and Fereidoun Azizi. "Complementary and alternative medicinal effects of broccoli sprouts powder on Helicobacter pylori eradication rate in type 2 diabetic patients: A randomized clinical trial." *Journal of Functional Foods* 7 (2014): 390-397.

47. Dang, Yini, Jan D. Reinhardt, Xiaoying Zhou, and Guoxin Zhang. "The effect of probiotics supplementation on Helicobacter pylori eradication rates and side effects during eradication therapy: a meta-analysis." *PloS one* 9, no. 11 (2014): e111030.

48. Song, Min Jun, Dong Il Park, Jung Ho Park, Hong Joo Kim, Yong Kyun Cho, Chong Il Sohn, Woo Kyu Jeon, and Byung Ik Kim. "The Effect of Probiotics and Mucoprotective Agents on PPI-Based Triple Therapy for Eradication of Helicobacter pylori." *Helicobacter* 15, no. 3 (2010): 206-213.

49. Lammers, Karen M., Ruliang Lu, Julie Brownley, Bao Lu, Craig Gerard, Karen Thomas, Prasad Rallabhandi et al. "Gliadin induces an increase in intestinal permeability and zonulin release by binding to the chemokine receptor CXCR3." *Gastroenterology* 135, no. 1 (2008): 194-204.

50. Longo, N. "Love Ice Cream? Here's how to make your own healthy varieties and avoid toxic ingredients." http://preventdisease.com/news/14/050714_Love-Ice-Cream-Heres-How-To-Make-Your-Own-Health-Varieties-Avoid-Toxic-Ingredients.shtml (Accessed February 2, 2016).

51. Behie, Alison M., Mary SM Pavelka, and Colin A. Chapman. "Sources of variation in fecal cortisol levels in howler monkeys in Belize." *American Journal of Primatology* 72, no. 7 (2010): 600-606.

52. Ulrich-Lai, Yvonne M., Michelle M. Ostrander, and James P. Herman. "HPA axis dampening by limited sucrose intake: reward frequency vs. caloric consumption." *Physiology & behavior* 103, no. 1 (2011): 104-110.

53. Niknahad, Hossein, Sumsullah Khan, Christian Sood, and Peter J. Obrien. "Prevention of cyanide-induced cytotoxicity by nutrients in isolated rat hepatocytes." *Toxicology and applied pharmacology* 128, no. 2 (1994): 271-279.

54. Niknahad, Hossein, Sumsullah Khan, and Peter J. O'Brien. "Hepatocyte injury resulting from the inhibition of mitochondrial respiration at low oxygen concentrations involves reductive stress and oxygen activation." *Chemico-biological interactions* 98, no. 1 (1995): 27-44.

55. Katoh, Kazuo, Mami Asari, Hiroko Ishiwata, Yasuyuki Sasaki, and Yoshiaki Obara. "Saturated fatty acids suppress adrenocorticotropic hormone (ACTH) release from rat anterior pituitary cells in vitro." *Comparative Biochemistry and Physiology Part A: Molecular & Integrative Physiology* 137, no. 2 (2004): 357-364.

56. Kirpich, Irina A., Wenke Feng, Yuhua Wang, Yanlong Liu, David F. Barker, Shirish S. Barve, and Craig J. McClain. "The Type of Dietary Fat Modulates Intestinal

Tight Junction Integrity, Gut Permeability, and Hepatic Toll-Like Receptor Expression in a Mouse Model of Alcoholic Liver Disease." *Alcoholism: Clinical and Experimental Research* 36, no. 5 (2012): 835-846.

57. Siebecker, Allison. "Traditional bone broth in modern health and disease." http://www.taylorwellness.com/wp-content/uploads/2012/11/Traditional-Bone-Broth-Siebecker.pdf (Accessed February 7, 2016).

58. Park, Y. W. "Hypo-allergenic and therapeutic significance of goat milk." *Small Ruminant Research* 14, no. 2 (1994): 151-159.

59. Kresser, Chris. "Raw Milk Reality: Benefits of Raw Milk." http://chriskresser.com/raw-milk-reality-benefits-of-raw-milk, (Accessed on March 2, 2016).

60. Jianqin, Sun, Xu Leiming, Xia Lu, Gregory W. Yelland Jiayi Ni, and Andrew J. Clarke. "Effects of milk containing only A2 beta casein versus milk containing both A1 and A2 beta casein proteins on gastrointestinal physiology, symptoms of discomfort, and cognitive behavior of people with self-reported intolerance to traditional cows' milk." *Nutrition journal* 15, no. 1 (2016): 35.

61. Amarowicz, Ryszard, Gary A. Dykes, and Ronald B. Pegg. "Antibacterial activity of tannin constituents from Phaseolus vulgaris, Fagoypyrum esculentum, Corylus

avellana and Juglans nigra." *Fitoterapia* 79, no. 3 (2008): 217-219.

62. Belknap, J. K., S. Giguere, A. Pettigrew, A. M. Cochran, AWv Eps, and C. C. Pollitt. "Lamellar pro-inflammatory cytokine expression patterns in laminitis at the developmental stage and at the onset of lameness: innate vs. adaptive immune response." *Equine veterinary journal* 39, no. 1 (2007): 42-47.

63. Bhargava, Umesh C., and Bertis A. Westfall. "Antitumor activity of Juglans nigra (black walnut) extractives." *Journal of pharmaceutical sciences* 57, no. 10 (1968): 1674-1677.

64. Park, Byeoung-Soo, Jun-Ran Kim, Sung-Eun Lee, Kyoung Soon Kim, Gary R. Takeoka, Young-Joon Ahn, and Jeong-Han Kim. "Selective growth-inhibiting effects of compounds identified in Tabebuia impetiginosa inner bark on human intestinal bacteria." *Journal of agricultural and food chemistry* 53, no. 4 (2005): 1152-1157.

65. Park, Byeoung-Soo, Hyun-Kyung Lee, Sung-Eun Lee, Xiang-Lan Piao, Gary R. Takeoka, Rosalind Y. Wong, Young-Joon Ahn, and Jeong-Han Kim. "Antibacterial activity of Tabebuia impetiginosa Martius ex DC (Taheebo) against Helicobacter pylori." *Journal of ethnopharmacology* 105, no. 1 (2006): 255-262.

66. Park, Byeoung-Soo, Kwang-Geun Lee, Takayuki Shibamoto, Sung-Eun Lee, and Gary R. Takeoka. "Antioxidant activity and characterization of volatile constituents of Taheebo (Tabebuia impetiginosa Martius ex DC)." *Journal of agricultural and food chemistry* 51, no. 1 (2003): 295-300.

67. Kim, Sung Ok, Jae Im Kwon, Yong Kee Jeong, Gi Young Kim, Nam Deuk Kim, and Yung Hyun Choi. "Induction of Egr-1 is associated with anti-metastatic and anti-invasive ability of β-lapachone in human hepatocarcinoma cells." *Bioscience, biotechnology, and biochemistry* 71, no. 9 (2007): 2169-2176.

68. Kung, Hsiu-Ni, Mei-Jun Yang, Chi-Fen Chang, Yat-Pang Chau, and Kuo-Shyan Lu. "In vitro and in vivo wound healing-promoting activities of β-lapachone." *American Journal of Physiology-Cell Physiology* 295, no. 4 (2008): C931-C943.

69. Taussig, Steven J., and Stanley Batkin. "Bromelain, the enzyme complex of pineapple (Ananas comosus) and its clinical application. An update." *Journal of ethnopharmacology* 22, no. 2 (1988): 191-203.

70. Kelly, Gregory S. "Bromelain: a literature review and discussion of its therapeutic applications." In *Alternative Medicine Review*. 1996.

71. Tomita, Mamoru, Wayne Bellamy, Mitsunori Takase, Koji Yamauchi, Hiroyuki Wakabayashi, and Kouzou Kawase.

"Potent antibacterial peptides generated by pepsin digestion of bovine lactoferrin." *Journal of Dairy Science* 74, no. 12 (1991): 4137-4142.

72. Butterworth, Peter J., Frederick J. Warren, and Peter R. Ellis. "Human α-amylase and starch digestion: An interesting marriage." *Starch-Stärke* 63, no. 7 (2011): 395-405.

73. Zimmermann, Robert, Juliane G. Strauss, Guenter Haemmerle, Gabriele Schoiswohl, Ruth Birner-Gruenberger, Monika Riederer, Achim Lass et al. "Fat mobilization in adipose tissue is promoted by adipose triglyceride lipase." *Science* 306, no. 5700 (2004): 1383-1386.

74. Cellulase http://worldofenzymes.info/enzymes-introduction/cellulase/ [Accessed March 5th, 2016].

75. World of Enzymes and Probiotics. "Invertase." http://worldofenzymes.info/enzymes-introduction/invertase/ (Accessed March 5, 2016).

76. Mercola, Joseph. "The Type of Food that Will Slow Nearly Every Inflammatory Disease." http://articles.mercola.com/sites/articles/archive/2011/08/21/enzymes-special-report.aspx (Accessed March 5, 2016).

77. Little, Katherine H., Lawrence R. Schiller, Lyman E. Bilhartz, and John S. Fordtran. "Treatment of severe steatorrhea with ox bile in an ileectomy patient with

residual colon." *Digestive diseases and sciences* 37, no. 6 (1992): 929-933.

78. McFarland Lynne V., and Sascha Dublin. "Meta-analysis of probiotics for the treatment of irritable bowel syndrome." *World journal of gastroenterology* 14, no. 17 (2008): 2650.

79. Yu, Zhihui, Xue Zhang, Shengyu Li, Changying Li, Da Li, and Zhennai Yang. "Evaluation of probiotic properties of Lactobacillus plantarum strains isolated from Chinese sauerkraut." *World Journal of Microbiology and Biotechnology* 29, no. 3 (2013): 489-498.

80. Duffy, L. C., M. A. Zielezny, M. Riepenhoff-Talty, D. Dryja, S. Sayahtaheri-Altaie, E. Griffiths, D. Ruffin, H. Barrett, J. Rossman, and P. L. Ogra. "Effectiveness of Bifidobacterium bifidum in mediating the clinical course of murine rotavirus diarrhea." *Pediatric research* 35, no. 6 (1994): 690-695.

81. Spanhaak, S., R. Havenaar, and G. Schaafsma. "The effect of consumption of milk fermented by Lactobacillus casei strain Shirota on the intestinal microflora and immune parameters in humans." *European Journal of Clinical Nutrition* 52, no. 12 (1998): 899-907.

82. Prebiotin. "Probiotics and stomach acid." https://www.prebiotin.com/probiotics-and-stomach-acid/ (Accessed April 4, 2016).

83. Kombucha. "What is kambucha?"
https://kombuchaforlife.wordpress.com/2013/05/15/what-is-kambucha/ (Accessed April 4, 2016).

84. Van Der Hulst, Rene RWJ, M. F. Von Meyenfeldt, N. E. P. Deutz, P. B. Soeters, R. J. M. Brummer, B. K. von Kreel, and J. W. Arends. "Glutamine and the preservation of gut integrity." *The Lancet* 341, no. 8857 (1993): 1363-1365.

85. Song, Qing-Hua, Rong-Mei Xu, Quan-Hai Zhang, Guo-Qing Shen, Ming Ma, Xin-Ping Zhao, Yan-Hua Guo, and Yi Wang. "Glutamine supplementation and immune function during heavy load training." *International journal of clinical pharmacology and therapeutics* 53, no. 5 (2015): 372-376.

86. Ewees, Mohamed Gamal, Basim Anwar Shehata Messiha, Ali Ahmed Abo-Saif, and Hekma Abd El-Tawab Abd El. "Is Coenzyme Q10 Effective in Protection against Ulcerative Colitis? An Experimental Study in Rats." *Biological and Pharmaceutical Bulletin* 39, no. 7 (2016): 1159-1166.

Chapter 3: The Hormone Trio and Your Thyroid

1. Wentz, I, Nowosadzka, M, *Hashimoto's Thyroiditis, Lifestyle Interventions for Finding and Treating the Root Cause*. (Wentz, LLC, 2013), 128-130.

2. Kazzarhian, Datis. *Why Do I Still Have Thyroid Symptoms?* (Carlsbad: Elephant Press,2010), 53-56.

3. Lerner, Aaron, Patricia Jeremias, and Torsten Matthias. "The world incidence and prevalence of autoimmune diseases is increasing." *International Journal of Celiac Disease* 3, no. 4 (2015): 151-155.

4. Holick, Michael F. "Vitamin D deficiency." *New England Journal of Medicine* 357, no. 3 (2007): 266-281.

5. Kamen, Diane L., and Vin Tangpricha. "Vitamin D and molecular actions on the immune system: modulation of innate and autoimmunity." *Journal of Molecular Medicine* 88, no. 5 (2010): 441-450.

6. Cantorna, Margherita T., and Brett D. Mahon. "Mounting evidence for vitamin D as an environmental factor affecting autoimmune disease prevalence." *Experimental biology and medicine* 229, no. 11 (2004): 1136-1142.

7. Holick, Michael F. "Sunlight and vitamin D." *Journal of General Internal Medicine* 17, no. 9 (2002): 733-735.

8. Holick, M.F., *The Vitamin D Solution – A 3 Step Strategy to Cure Our Most Common Health Problems*. (New York: Penguin, 2010) 217.

9. Simopoulos, Artemis P. "Omega-3 fatty acids in inflammation and autoimmune diseases." *Journal of the American College of Nutrition* 21, no. 6 (2002): 495-505.

10. Harding, Anne. "Low-FODMAP Diet Shifts Metabolome, Microbiome in IBS Patients." http://www.medscape.com/viewarticle/861280 (Accessed May 1st, 2016)

11. Sun, Jia, Laetitia Furio, Ramine Mecheri, Anne M. van der Does, Erik Lundeberg, Loredana Saveanu, Yongquan Chen, Peter van Endert, Birgitta Agerberth, and Julien Diana. "Pancreatic β-cells limit autoimmune diabetes via an immunoregulatory antimicrobial peptide expressed under the influence of the gut microbiota." *Immunity* 43, no. 2 (2015): 304-317.

12. Smecuol, Edgardo, Hui J. Hwang, Emilia Sugai, Laura Corso, Alejandra C. Cherñavsky, Franco P. Bellavite, Andrea González et al. "Exploratory, randomized, double-blind, placebo-controlled study on the effects of Bifidobacterium infantis natren life start strain super strain in active celiac disease." *Journal of clinical gastroenterology* 47, no. 2 (2013): 139-147.

13. Jimenez, Claudia, Irene Leets, Rafael Puche, Elsy Anzola, Rosa Montilla, Cesar Parra, Antonia Aguilera, and María N. García-Casal. "A single dose of vitamin A improves haemoglobin concentration, retinol status and phagocytic

function of neutrophils in preschool children." *British Journal of Nutrition* 103, no. 06 (2010): 798-802..

14. Muñoz, Elsa C., Jorge L. Rosado, Patricia López, Harold C. Furr, and Lindsay H. Allen. "Iron and zinc supplementation improves indicators of vitamin A status of Mexican preschoolers." *The American journal of clinical nutrition* 71, no. 3 (2000): 789-794.

15. Ahsan, Haseeb, Amjid Ahad, Jahangir Iqbal, and Waseem A. Siddiqui. "Pharmacological potential of tocotrienols: a review." *Nutrition & metabolism* 11, no. 1 (2014): 52.

16. Qureshi, Asaf A., Huanbiao Mo, Lester Packer, and David M. Peterson. "Isolation and identification of novel tocotrienols from rice bran with hypocholesterolemic, antioxidant, and antitumor properties." *Journal of Agricultural and Food Chemistry* 48, no. 8 (2000): 3130-3140.

17. Tan, Barrie, and Linda Brzuskiewicz. "Separation of tocopherol and tocotrienol isomers using normal-and reverse-phase liquid chromatography." *Analytical biochemistry* 180, no. 2 (1989): 368-373.

18. Aggarwal, Bharat B., Chitra Sundaram, Seema Prasad, and Ramaswamy Kannappan. "Tocotrienols, the vitamin E of the 21st century: its potential against cancer and other chronic diseases." *Biochemical pharmacology* 80, no. 11 (2010): 1613-1631.

19. Ng, S. C., Y. T. Lam, K. K. F. Tsoi, F. K. L. Chan, J. J. Y. Sung, and J. C. Y. Wu. "Systematic review: the efficacy of herbal therapy in inflammatory bowel disease." *Alimentary pharmacology & therapeutics* 38, no. 8 (2013): 854-863.

20. Gupta, Subash C., Sridevi Patchva, and Bharat B. Aggarwal. "Therapeutic roles of curcumin: lessons learned from clinical trials." *The AAPS journal* 15, no. 1 (2013): 195-218.

21. Larmo, P., J. Alin, E. Salminen, H. Kallio, and R. Tahvonen. "Effects of sea buckthorn berries on infections and inflammation: a double-blind, randomized, placebo-controlled trial." *European journal of clinical nutrition* 62, no. 9 (2008): 1123-1130.

22. De Palma, Giada, Inmaculada Nadal, Maria Carmen Collado, and Yolanda Sanz. "Effects of a gluten-free diet on gut microbiota and immune function in healthy adult human subjects." *British Journal of Nutrition* 102, no. 08 (2009): 1154-1160.

23. Kresser, Chris. "Five ways that stress causes hypothyroid symptoms." http://chriskresser.com/5-ways-that-stress-causes-hypothyroid-symptoms/ (Accessed May 3, 2016).

24. Walter, Kimberly N., Elizabeth J. Corwin, Jan Ulbrecht, Laurence M. Demers, Jeanette M. Bennett, Courtney A. Whetzel, and Laura Cousino Klein. "Elevated thyroid

stimulating hormone is associated with elevated cortisol in healthy young men and women." *Thyroid research* 5, no. 1 (2012): 13.

25. Zeng, Yawen, Jiazhen Yang, Juan Du, Xiaoying Pu, Xiaomen Yang, Shuming Yang, and Tao Yang. "Strategies of functional foods promote sleep in human being." *Current signal transduction therapy* 9, no. 3 (2014): 148-155.

26. Yang, Mihi, Ho-Sun Lee, Min-Woo Hwang, and Mirim Jin. "Effects of Korean red ginseng (Panax Ginseng Meyer) on bisphenol A exposure and gynecologic complaints: single blind, randomized clinical trial of efficacy and safety." *BMC complementary and alternative medicine* 14, no. 1 (2014): 265.

27. Cui, Xiang-Yu, Su-Ying Cui, Juan Zhang, Zi-Jun Wang, Bin Yu, Zhao-Fu Sheng, Xue-Qiong Zhang, and Yong-He Zhang. "Extract of Ganoderma lucidum prolongs sleep time in rats." *Journal of ethnopharmacology* 139, no. 3 (2012): 796-800.

28. Kruger, Allison K., Eric N. Reither, Paul E. Peppard, Patrick M. Krueger, and Lauren Hale. "Do sleep-deprived adolescents make less-healthy food choices?." *British Journal of Nutrition* 111, no. 10 (2014): 1898-1904.

29. Katagiri, Ryoko, Keiko Asakura, Satomi Kobayashi, Hitomi Suga, and Satoshi Sasaki. "Low intake of vegetables, high intake of confectionary, and unhealthy

eating habits are associated with poor sleep quality among middle-aged female Japanese workers." *Journal of occupational health* 56, no. 5 (2014): 359-368.

30. Zeng, Yawen, Jiazhen Yang, Juan Du, Xiaoying Pu, Xiaomen Yang, Shuming Yang, and Tao Yang. "Strategies of functional foods promote sleep in human being." *Current signal transduction therapy* 9, no. 3 (2014): 148-155.

31. Kota, Sunil Kumar, Lalit Kumar Meher, S. V. S. Krishna, and K. D. Modi. "Hypothyroidism in metabolic syndrome." *Indian Journal of Endocrinology & Metabolism* 16 (2012).

32. Attele, Anoja S., Yun-Ping Zhou, Jing-Tian Xie, Ji An Wu, Liu Zhang, Lucy Dey, William Pugh, Paul A. Rue, Kenneth S. Polonsky, and Chun-Su Yuan. "Antidiabetic effects of Panax ginseng berry extract and the identification of an effective component." *Diabetes* 51, no. 6 (2002): 1851-1858.

33. Methlie, Paal, Eystein ES Husebye, Steinar Hustad, Ernst A. Lien, and Kristian Løvås. "Grapefruit juice and licorice increase cortisol availability in patients with Addison's disease." *European journal of endocrinology* 165, no. 5 (2011): 761-769.

34. Provino, Robert. "The role of adaptogens in stress management." *Australian Journal of Medical Herbalism* 22, no. 2 (2010): 41.

35. Bhattacharya, S. K., A. Bhattacharya, K. Sairam, and S. Ghosal. "Anxiolytic-antidepressant activity of Withania somnifera glycowithanolides: an experimental study." *Phytomedicine* 7, no. 6 (2000): 463-469.

36. Gannon, Jessica M., Paige E. Forrest, and KN Roy Chengappa. "Subtle changes in thyroid indices during a placebo-controlled study of an extract of Withania somnifera in persons with bipolar disorder." *Journal of Ayurveda and integrative medicine* 5, no. 4 (2014): 241.

37. Jothie Richard, Edwin, Ramanaiah Illuri, Bharathi Bethapudi, Senthilkumar Anandhakumar, Anirban Bhaskar, Chandrasekaran Chinampudur Velusami, Deepak Mundkinajeddu, and Amit Agarwal. "Anti-stress Activity of Ocimum sanctum: Possible Effects on Hypothalamic–Pituitary–Adrenal Axis." *Phytotherapy Research* (2016).

38. Examine. "Rhodiola rosea." https://examine.com/supplements/rhodiola-rosea/#citations (Accessed July5, 2016).

39. Talbott, Shawn. "The Cortisol connection, Chapter 8." http://cortisolconnection.com/ch8_6.php (Accessed July 5, 2016).

40. Rizk, Jacqueline. "Hormonal imbalance? Think thyroid!" www.thedetoxdiva.com/hormonal-imbalance-think-thyroid/ (Accessed July 5, 2016).

41. Gottfried Sara. *The Hormone Cure*. (New York: Scribner, 2013)

42. Phelan, Niamh, Annalouise O'Connor, Tommy Kyaw Tun, Neuman Correia, Gerard Boran, Helen M. Roche, and James Gibney. "Hormonal and metabolic effects of polyunsaturated fatty acids in young women with polycystic ovary syndrome: results from a cross-sectional analysis and a randomized, placebo-controlled, crossover trial." *The American journal of clinical nutrition* 93, no. 3 (2011): 652-662.

Chapter 4: Foods and Environmental Factors that Affect Thyroid Function Negatively

1. Sategna-Guidetti, C., U. Volta, C. Ciacci, P. Usai, A. Carlino, L. De Franceschi, A. Camera, A. Pelli, and C. Brossa. "Prevalence of thyroid disorders in untreated adult celiac disease patients and effect of gluten withdrawal: an Italian multicenter study." The American journal of gastroenterology 96, no. 3 (2001): 751-757.

2. Drago, Sandro, Ramzi El Asmar, Mariarosaria Di Pierro, Maria Grazia Clemente, Amit Tripathi Anna Sapone, Manjusha Thakar, Giuseppe Iacono et al. "Gliadin, zonulin and gut permeability: Effects on celiac and non-celiac intestinal mucosa and intestinal cell lines." Scandinavian journal of gastroenterology 41, no. 4 (2006): 408-419.

3. Nadhem, Omar N., Ghassan Azeez, Roger D. Smalligan, and Steven Urban. "Review and practice guidelines for celiac disease in 2014." Postgraduate medicine 127, no. 3 (2015): 259-265.

4. Molina-Infante, J., S. Santolaria, D. S. Sanders, and F. Fernández-Bañares. "Systematic review: noncoeliac gluten sensitivity." Alimentary pharmacology & therapeutics 41, no. 9 (2015): 807-820.

5. Fan, Ming-Sheng, Fang-Jie Zhao, Susan J. Fairweather-Tait, Paul R. Poulton, Sarah J. Dunham, and Steve P. McGrath. "Evidence of decreasing mineral density in wheat grain over the last 160 years." *Journal of Trace*

Elements in Medicine and Biology 22, no. 4 (2008): 315-324.

6. Zhao, F. J., Y. H. Su, S. J. Dunham, M. Rakszegi, Z. Bedo, S. P. McGrath, and P. R. Shewry. "Variation in mineral micronutrient concentrations in grain of wheat lines of diverse origin." *Journal of Cereal Science* 49, no. 2 (2009): 290-295.

7. Van den Broeck, Hetty C., Hein C. de Jong, Elma MJ Salentijn, Liesbeth Dekking, Dirk Bosch, Rob J. Hamer, Ludovicus JWJ Gilissen, Ingrid M. van der Meer, and Marinus JM Smulders. "Presence of celiac disease epitopes in modern and old hexaploid wheat varieties: wheat breeding may have contributed to increased prevalence of celiac disease." *Theoretical and Applied Genetics* 121, no. 8 (2010): 1527-1539.

8. Pizzuti, Daniela, Andrea Buda, Anna d'Odorico, Renata d'Incà, Silvia Chiarelli, Andrea Curioni, and Diego Martines. "Lack of intestinal mucosal toxicity of Triticum monococcum in celiac disease patients." *Scandinavian journal of gastroenterology* 41, no. 11 (2006): 1305-1311.

9. Sofi, Francesco, A. Whittaker, F. Cesari, Anna Maria Gori, C. Fiorillo, M. Becatti, I. Marotti et al. "Characterization of Khorasan wheat (Kamut) and impact of a replacement diet on cardiovascular risk factors: cross-

over dietary intervention study." *European journal of clinical nutrition* 67, no. 2 (2013): 190-195.

10. Saa, Danielle Taneyo, Silvia Turroni, Diana Isabella Serrazanetti, Simone Rampelli, Simone Maccaferri, Marco Candela, Marco Severgnini, Emanuela Simonetti, Patrizia Brigidi, and Andrea Gianotti. "Impact of Kamut® Khorasan on gut microbiota and metabolome in healthy volunteers." *Food Research International* 63 (2014): 227-232.

11. Parameswaran, K. Parvathy, and S. Sadasivam. "Changes in the carbohydrates and nitrogenous components during germination of proso millet, Panicum miliaceum." *Plant Foods for Human Nutrition* 45, no. 2 (1994): 97-102.

12. Koehler, Peter, Georg Hartmann, Herbert Wieser, and Michael Rychlik. "Changes of folates, dietary fiber, and proteins in wheat as affected by germination." *Journal of agricultural and food chemistry* 55, no. 12 (2007): 4678-4683.

13. Di Cagno, Raffaella, Maria De Angelis, Salvatore Auricchio, Luigi Greco, Charmaine Clarke, Massimo De Vincenzi, Claudio Giovannini et al. "Sourdough bread made from wheat and nontoxic flours and started with selected lactobacilli is tolerated in celiac sprue patients." *Applied and environmental microbiology* 70, no. 2 (2004): 1088-1096.

14. Chassaing, Benoit, Omry Koren, Julia K. Goodrich, Angela C. Poole, Shanthi Srinivasan, Ruth E. Ley, and Andrew T. Gewirtz. "Dietary emulsifiers impact the mouse gut microbiota promoting colitis and metabolic syndrome." *Nature* 519, no. 7541 (2015): 92-96.

15. Kresser, Chris. "The Gluten-Thyroid Connection." https://chriskresser.com/the-gluten-thyroid-connection/ (Accessed August, 2016).

16. Divi, Rao L., and Daniel R. Doerge. "Inhibition of thyroid peroxidase by dietary flavonoids." *Chemical research in toxicology* 9, no. 1 (1996): 16-23.

17. Fruzza, Abigail Gelb, Carla Demeterco-Berggren, and Kenneth Lee Jones. "Unawareness of the effects of soy intake on the management of congenital hypothyroidism." *Pediatrics* 130, no. 3 (2012): e699-e702.

18. Shapiro, Theresa A., Jed W. Fahey, Albena T. Dinkova-Kostova, W. David Holtzclaw, Katherine K. Stephenson, Kristina L. Wade, Lingxiang Ye, and Paul Talalay. "Safety, tolerance, and metabolism of broccoli sprout glucosinolates and isothiocyanates: a clinical phase I study." *Nutrition and cancer* 55, no. 1 (2006): 53-62.

19. Chandler, Joshua D., and Brian J. Day. "Thiocyanate: a potentially useful therapeutic agent with host defense and antioxidant properties." *Biochemical pharmacology* 84, no. 11 (2012): 1381-1387.

20. Medline Plus. "Vitamin B12 deficiency anemia." https://www.nlm.nih.gov/medlineplus/ency/article/000574 .htm (Accessed May 2, 2016).

21. Zhu, Yingying, Xisha Lin, Fan Zhao, Xuebin Shi, He Li, Yingqiu Li, Weiyun Zhu, Xinglian Xu, Chunbao Li, and Guanghong Zhou. "Meat, dairy and plant proteins alter bacterial composition of rat gut bacteria." *Scientific reports* 5 (2015): 15220.

22. Step to Health. "Eight household products that can affect the thyroid." http://steptohealth.com/eight-household-products-can-affect-thyroid/ (Accessed October 22, 2016).

23. Ballantyne, Sarah, *The Paleo Approach, Reverse Autoimmune Disease and Heal Your Body*. (Las Vegas: Victory Belt Publishing Inc., 2013)

Chapter 5: Diets and Foods to Consider for Hypothyroidism

1. Cole, William. "Eleven everyday toxins that are harming your thyroid." http://www.mindbodygreen.com/0-12346/11-everyday-toxins-that-are-harming-your-thyroid.html (Accessed February 4, 2016).

2. Carahealth. "Phase 1 and 2 Liver Detoxification Pathways." http://www.carahealth.com/health-conditions-a-to-z/digestive-system/detox/365-phase-1-and-2-liver-detoxification-pathways60.html (Accessed February 7, 2016).

3. Flora, Kenneth, Martin Hahn, Hugo Rosen, and Kent Benner. "Milk thistle (Silybum marianum) for the therapy of liver disease." *The American journal of gastroenterology* 93, no. 2 (1998): 139-143.

4. Kazzarhian, Datis. *Why Do I Still Have Thyroid Symptoms?* (Carlsbad: Elephant Press,2010).

5. Sekhar, Rajagopal V., Sanjeet G. Patel, Anuradha P. Guthikonda, Marvin Reid, Ashok Balasubramanyam, George E. Taffet, and Farook Jahoor. "Deficient synthesis of glutathione underlies oxidative stress in aging and can be corrected by dietary cysteine and glycine supplementation." *The American journal of clinical nutrition* 94, no. 3 (2011): 847-853.

6. Ottenberg, Reuben. "Painless jaundice." *Journal of the American Medical Association* 104, no. 19 (1935): 1681-1688.

7. Environmental Working Group. "Clean Fifteen." https://www.ewg.org/foodnews/clean_fifteen_list.php (Accessed February 10, 2016).

8. "10 Reasons to Use a Water Filter." http://www.allaboutwater.org/water-filter.html (Accessed March 1, 2016).

9. Siri-Tarino, Patty W., Qi Sun, Frank B. Hu, and Ronald M. Krauss. "Meta-analysis of prospective cohort studies evaluating the association of saturated fat with cardiovascular disease." *The American journal of clinical nutrition* (2010): ajcn-27725.

10. Enig, Mary. "Fats and Oils and Their Impact on Health." http://www.westonaprice.org/health-topics/fats-and-oils-and-their-impact-on-health/#sthash.ZcbBb6xw.dpuf (Accessed March 2, 2016).

11. Legrand Philippe, and Vincent Rioux. "The complex and important cellular and metabolic functions of saturated fatty acids." *Lipids* 45, no. 10 (2010): 941-946.

12. Legrand P. "Origin, metabolism and biological functions of saturated fatty acids." http://www.aocs.org/files/resourcespdf/legrand-aocs-orlando-09-transmis.pdf. (Accessed March 2, 2016).

13. Enig, Mary. "The Importance of Saturated Fats for Biological Functions." https://www.westonaprice.org/health-topics/know-your-fats/the-importance-of-saturated-fats-for-biological-functions/ (Accessed March 2, 2016).

14. Mercola, Joseph. "Seven Reasons to Eat More Saturated Fat." http://articles.mercola.com/sites/articles/archive/2009/09/2 2/7-reasons-to-eat-more-saturated-fat.aspx (Accessed March 2, 2016).

15. Micha, Renata, and Dariush Mozaffarian. "Saturated fat and cardiometabolic risk factors, coronary heart disease, stroke, and diabetes: a fresh look at the evidence." *Lipids* 45, no. 10 (2010): 893-905.

16. Ramsden, Christopher E., Daisy Zamora, Boonseng Leelarthaepin, Sharon F. Majchrzak-Hong, Keturah R. Faurot, Chirayath M. Suchindran, Amit Ringel, John M. Davis, and Joseph R. Hibbeln. "Use of dietary linoleic acid for secondary prevention of coronary heart disease and death: evaluation of recovered data from the Sydney Diet Heart Study and updated meta-analysis." *Bmj* 346 (2013): e8707.

17. Friedlander, Jodi. "Saturated fats: Separating Myth from Fact." http://www.baumancollege.org/blog/saturated-fats-myths-and-facts (Accessed March 10, 2016).

18. Miller, D.W. "Enjoy saturated fats, they're good for you!" http://lewrockwell.com/miller/miller38.1.html. (Accessed March 10, 2016).

19. Chevaux, Kati A., Lilian Jackson, Maria Elena Villar, Jeff A. Mundt, Joel F. Commisso, Gary E. Adamson, Marjorie M. McCullough, Harold H. Schmitz, and Norman K. Hollenberg. "Proximate, mineral and procyanidin content of certain foods and beverages consumed by the Kuna Amerinds of Panama." *Journal of food composition and analysis* 14, no. 6 (2001): 553-563.

20. Rein, Dietrich, Teresa G. Paglieroni, Ted Wun, Debra A. Pearson, Harold H. Schmitz, Robert Gosselin, and Carl L. Keen. "Cocoa inhibits platelet activation and function." *The American journal of clinical nutrition* 72, no. 1 (2000): 30-35.

21. Waterhouse, Andrew L., Joseph R. Shirley, and Jennifer L. Donovan. "Antioxidants in chocolate." *The Lancet* 348, no. 9030 (1996): 834.

22. Säemann, Marcus D., Georg A. Böhmig, Christoph H. Österreicher, Helmut Burtscher, Ornella Parolini, Christos Diakos, Johannes Stöckl, Walter H. Hörl, and Gerhard J. Zlabinger. "Anti-inflammatory effects of sodium butyrate on human monocytes: potent inhibition of IL-12 and up-regulation of IL-10 production." *The FASEB Journal* 14, no. 15 (2000): 2380-2382.

23. Nishii Y., et al. "n-Butyrate enhances induction of thyroid hormone-responsive nuclear protein." *Endocrine Journal.* 40, no.5 (1993): 515-521.

24. Hamer, Henrike M., D. M. A. E. Jonkers, Koen Venema, S. A. L. W. Vanhoutvin, F. J. Troost, and R-J. Brummer. "Review article: the role of butyrate on colonic function." *Alimentary pharmacology & therapeutics* 27, no. 2 (2008): 104-119.

25. Lührs, H., T. Gerke, J. G. Müller, R. Melcher, J. Schauber, F. Boxberger, W. Scheppach, and T. Menzel. "Butyrate inhibits NF-κB activation in lamina propria macrophages of patients with ulcerative colitis." *Scandinavian journal of gastroenterology* 37, no. 4 (2002): 458-466.

26. Lührs, H., T. Gerke, J. G. Müller, R. Melcher, J. Schauber, F. Boxberger, W. Scheppach, and T. Menzel. "Butyrate inhibits NF-κB activation in lamina propria macrophages of patients with ulcerative colitis." *Scandinavian journal of gastroenterology* 37, no. 4 (2002): 458-466.

27. Vermeer, Cees, Martin J. Shearer, Armin Zittermann, Caroline Bolton-Smith, Pawel Szulc, Stephen Hodges, Paul Walter, Walter Rambeck, Elisabeth Stöcklin, and Peter Weber. "Beyond deficiency." *European journal of nutrition* 43, no. 6 (2004): 325-335.

28. Geleijnse, Johanna M., Cees Vermeer, Diederick E. Grobbee, Leon J. Schurgers, Marjo HJ Knapen, Irene M.

Van Der Meer, Albert Hofman, and Jacqueline CM Witteman. "Dietary intake of menaquinone is associated with a reduced risk of coronary heart disease: the Rotterdam Study." *The Journal of nutrition* 134, no. 11 (2004): 3100-3105.

29. Gast, Gerrie-Cor M., Nicole M. de Roos, Ivonne Sluijs, Michiel L. Bots, Joline WJ Beulens, Johanna M. Geleijnse, Jacqueline C. Witteman, Diederick E. Grobbee, Petra HM Peeters, and Yvonne T. van der Schouw. "A high menaquinone intake reduces the incidence of coronary heart disease." *Nutrition, Metabolism and Cardiovascular Diseases* 19, no. 7 (2009): 504-510.

30. Daley, Cynthia A., Amber Abbott, Patrick S. Doyle, Glenn A. Nader, and Stephanie Larson. "A review of fatty acid profiles and antioxidant content in grass-fed and grain-fed beef." *Nutrition journal* 9, no. 1 (2010): 10.

31. Traber, Maret G., and Jeffrey Atkinson. "Vitamin E, antioxidant and nothing more." *Free Radical Biology and Medicine* 43, no. 1 (2007): 4-15.

32. Kresser, Chris. "Why grass-fed trumps grain fed." http://chriskresser.com/why-grass-fed-trumps-grain-fed/ (Accessed May14, 2016).

33. Kabara, Jon J., Dennis M. Swieczkowski, Anthony J. Conley, and Joseph P. Truant. "Fatty acids and derivatives as antimicrobial agents." *Antimicrobial agents and chemotherapy* 2, no. 1 (1972): 23-28.

34. Ruzin, Alexey, and Richard P. Novick. "Equivalence of lauric acid and glycerol monolaurate as inhibitors of signal transduction in Staphylococcus aureus." *Journal of Bacteriology* 182, no. 9 (2000): 2668-2671.

35. Ogbolu, David Olusoga, Anthony Alaba Oni, Oluwole Adebayo Daini, and A. P. Oloko. "In vitro antimicrobial properties of coconut oil on Candida species in Ibadan, Nigeria." *Journal of medicinal food* 10, no. 2 (2007): 384-387.

36. Assunçao, Monica L., Haroldo S. Ferreira, Aldenir F. dos Santos, Cyro R. Cabral, and Telma MMT Florêncio. "Effects of dietary coconut oil on the biochemical and anthropometric profiles of women presenting abdominal obesity." *Lipids* 44, no. 7 (2009): 593-601.

37. Liau, Kai Ming, Yeong Yeh Lee, Chee Keong Chen, and Aida Hanum G. Rasool. "An open-label pilot study to assess the efficacy and safety of virgin coconut oil in reducing visceral adiposity." *ISRN pharmacology* 2011 (2011).

38. Basu, Arpita, Sridevi Devaraj, and Ishwarlal Jialal. "Dietary factors that promote or retard inflammation." *Arteriosclerosis, thrombosis, and vascular biology* 26, no. 5 (2006): 995-1001.

39. Yoneyama, Satoko, Katsuyuki Miura, Satoshi Sasaki, Katsushi Yoshita, Yuko Morikawa, Masao Ishizaki,

Teruhiko Kido, Yuchi Naruse, and Hideaki Nakagawa. "Dietary intake of fatty acids and serum C-reactive protein in Japanese." *Journal of epidemiology* 17, no. 3 (2007): 86-92.

40. Lucas, Lisa, Aaron Russell, and Russell Keast. "Molecular mechanisms of inflammation. Anti-inflammatory benefits of virgin olive oil and the phenolic compound oleocanthal." *Current pharmaceutical design* 17, no. 8 (2011): 754-768.

41. Beauchamp, Gary K., Russell SJ Keast, Diane Morel, Jianming Lin, Jana Pika, Qiang Han, Chi-Ho Lee, Amos B. Smith, and Paul AS Breslin. "Phytochemistry: ibuprofen-like activity in extra-virgin olive oil." *Nature* 437, no. 7055 (2005): 45-46.

42. Hopkin, Michael. "Extra-virgin olive oils mimics painkiller." http://www.nature.com/news/2005/050829/full/news0508 29-11.html (Accessed April 7, 2016).

43. Anticancer. "Flaxseeds are useful and pose no danger to the thyroid." http://www.anticancerbook.com/post/Flax-seeds-are-useful-and-pose-no-danger-to-the-thyroid.html (Accessed April 7, 2016).

44. Axe, Josh. "10 Flax Seed Benefits and Nutrition Facts." http://draxe.com/10-flax-seed-benefits-nutrition-facts/ (Accessed April 7, 2016).

45. Mercola, Joseph. "This antioxidant can smash insulin resistance and autoimmune disease." http://articles.mercola.com/sites/articles/archive/2009/05/1 6/this-antioxidant-can-smash-insulin-resistance-and-autoimmune-disease.aspx (Accessed April 7, 2016).

46. Axe, Josh. "The Truth About Saturated Fat." http://draxe.com/the-truth-about-saturated-fat/ (Accessed April 7, 2016).

47. Simopoulos, Artemis P. "Omega-3 fatty acids in inflammation and autoimmune diseases." *Journal of the American College of Nutrition* 21, no. 6 (2002): 495-505.

48. Goldberg, Robert J., and Joel Katz. "A meta-analysis of the analgesic effects of omega-3 polyunsaturated fatty acid supplementation for inflammatory joint pain." *Pain* 129, no. 1 (2007): 210-223.

49. Souza, Luana L., Marcio O. Nunes, Gabriela SM Paula, Aline Cordeiro, Vânia Penha-Pinto, Jose Firmino N. Neto, Karen J. Oliveira, Maria das Graças Tavares do Carmo, and Carmen C. Pazos-Moura. "Effects of dietary fish oil on thyroid hormone signaling in the liver." *The Journal of nutritional biochemistry* 21, no. 10 (2010): 935-940.

50. Mueller, Kathryn. "Novel Diet Therapy Helps Children With Crohn's Disease and Ulcerative Colitis Reach Remission." http://pulse.seattlechildrens.org/novel-diet-therapy-helps-children-with-crohns-disease-and-

ulcerative-colitis-reach-remission/ (Accessed December 30, 2016).

51. Examples of food high in FODMAPs and suitable low FODMAP alternatives. https://www.ncbi.nlm.nih.gov/pmc/articles/PMC4918736/table/t2-ceg-9-131/ (Accessed October 8, 2016).

52. Nanayakkara, Wathsala S., Paula ML Skidmore, Leigh O'Brien, Tim J. Wilkinson, and Richard B. Gearry. "Efficacy of the low FODMAP diet for treating irritable bowel syndrome: the evidence to date." *Clinical and Experimental Gastroenterology* 9 (2016): 131.

53. Vandyken, Paul. "What to eat on the Paleo diet." http://thepaleodiet.com/what-to-eat-on-the-paleo-diet/ (Accessed October 8, 2016).

54. Manheimer, Eric W., Esther J. van Zuuren, Zbys Fedorowicz, and Hanno Pijl. "Paleolithic nutrition for metabolic syndrome: systematic review and meta-analysis." *The American journal of clinical nutrition* 102, no. 4 (2015): 922-932.

55. Adapted from: http://ultimatepaleoguide.com/autoimmune-protocol/ (Accessed October 8, 2016).

56. Vojdani, Aristo. "Lectins, agglutinins, and their roles in autoimmune reactivities." *health* 2 (2015): 4.

57. Ballantyne, Sarah, *The Paleo Approach, Reverse Autoimmune Disease and Heal Your Body*. (Las Vegas: Victory Belt Publishing Inc., 2013)

58. World Health Organization. "CALCIUM AND MAGNESIUM IN DRINKING WATER: PUBLIC HEALTH SIGNIFICANCE." (Accessed March 5, 2016).

59. Altura, Burton M., and Bella T. Altura. "Magnesium: forgotten mineral in cardiovascular biology and atherogenesis." In *New Perspectives in Magnesium Research*, pp. 239-260. Springer London, 2007.

60. Seelig, Mildred S., and Andrea Rosanoff. *The magnesium factor*. Penguin, 2003.

61. Thomas, David. "The Mineral Depletion of Foods Available to Us as a Nation (1940–2002)—A Review of the 6th Edition of MCance and Widdowson." *Nutrition and health* 19, no. 1-2 (2007): 21-55.

62. Ancient Minerals. "Symptoms of Low Magnesium." http://www.ancient-minerals.com/magnesium-deficiency/symptoms-signs/ (Accessed March 16, 2016).

63. Abbas, Amr M., and Hussein F. Sakr. "Effect of magnesium sulfate and thyroxine on inflammatory markers in a rat model of hypothyroidism." *Canadian journal of physiology and pharmacology* 94, no. 4 (2015): 426-432.

64. Simental-Mendía, Luis E., Amirhossein Sahebkar, Martha Rodríguez-Morán, and Fernando Guerrero-Romero. "A systematic review and meta-analysis of randomized controlled trials on the effects of magnesium supplementation on insulin sensitivity and glucose control." *Pharmacological research* 111 (2016): 272-282.

65. Betsy, Ambooken, M. P. Binitha, and S. Sarita. "Zinc deficiency associated with hypothyroidism: an overlooked cause of severe alopecia." *International journal of trichology* 5, no. 1 (2013): 40.

66. Alhaj, Eyad, Nehad Alhaj, and Nezam E. Alhaj. "Diffuse alopecia in a child due to dietary zinc deficiency." *SKINmed: Dermatology for the Clinician* 6, no. 4 (2007): 199-200.

67. Mayo Clinic. "Zinc." http://www.mayoclinic.org/drugs-supplements/zinc/dosing/hrb-20060638 (Accessed October 3, 2016).

68. Wegmüller, Rita, Fabian Tay, Christophe Zeder, Marica Brnić, and Richard F. Hurrell. "Zinc absorption by young adults from supplemental zinc citrate is comparable with that from zinc gluconate and higher than from zinc oxide." *The Journal of nutrition* 144, no. 2 (2014): 132-136.

69. Uauy, Ricardo, Manuel Olivares, and Mauricio Gonzalez. "Essentiality of copper in humans." *The American journal of clinical nutrition* 67, no. 5 (1998): 952S-959S.

70. Axe, Josh. "Top 10 Foods High in Selenium." https://draxe.com/top-10-foods-high-selenium/ (Accessed October 5, 2016).

71. Drutel, Anne, Françoise Archambeaud, and Philippe Caron. "Selenium and the thyroid gland: more good news for clinicians." *Clinical endocrinology* 78, no. 2 (2013): 155-164.

72. Duntas, L. H. "The role of iodine and selenium in autoimmune thyroiditis." *Hormone and Metabolic Research* 47, no. 10 (2015): 721-726.

73. Vasiliu I et al. "Selenium status in autoimmune thyroiditis." *Rev Med Chir Soc Med Nat Iasi* 119, no. 4 (2015): 1037-44.

74. de Farias, C. R., B. R. Cardoso, G. M. B. de Oliveira, I. C. de Mello Guazzelli, R. M. Catarino, M. C. Chammas, S. M. F. Cozzolino, and M. Knobel. "A randomized-controlled, double-blind study of the impact of selenium supplementation on thyroid autoimmunity and inflammation with focus on the GPx1 genotypes." *Journal of endocrinological investigation* 38, no. 10 (2015): 1065-1074.

75. Burk, Raymond F., Brooke K. Norsworthy, Kristina E. Hill, Amy K. Motley, and Daniel W. Byrne. "Effects of chemical form of selenium on plasma biomarkers in a high-dose human supplementation trial." *Cancer*

Epidemiology and Prevention Biomarkers 15, no. 4 (2006): 804-810.

76. Pedersen, Inge B., Nils Knudsen, Allan Carlé, Pernille Vejbjerg, Torben Jørgensen, Hans Perrild, Lars Ovesen, Lone B. Rasmussen, and Peter Laurberg. "A cautious iodization programme bringing iodine intake to a low recommended level is associated with an increase in the prevalence of thyroid autoantibodies in the population." *Clinical endocrinology* 75, no. 1 (2011): 120-126.

77. Camargo, Rosalinda YA, Eduardo K. Tomimori, Solange C. Neves, Ileana GS Rubio, Ana Luiza Galrão, Meyer Knobel, and Geraldo Medeiros-Neto. "Thyroid and the environment: exposure to excessive nutritional iodine increases the prevalence of thyroid disorders in Sao Paulo, Brazil." *European journal of endocrinology* 159, no. 3 (2008): 293-299.

78. Mayo Clinic. "Iron deficiency anemia." http://www.mayoclinic.org/diseases-conditions/iron-deficiency-anemia/basics/symptoms/con-20019327 (Accessed October 10, 2016).

79. Veltri, Flora, Sarah Decaillet, Pierre Kleynen, Lidia Grabczan, Julie Belhomme, Serge Rozenberg, Thierry Pepersack, and Kris Poppe. "Prevalence of thyroid autoimmunity and dysfunction in women with iron deficiency during early pregnancy: is it

altered?." *European Journal of Endocrinology* 175, no. 3 (2016): 191-199.

80. M'Rabet-Bensalah, Khadija, Carole E. Aubert, Michael Coslovsky, Tinh-Hai Collet, Christine Baumgartner, Wendy PJ Elzen, Robert Luben et al. "Thyroid dysfunction and anaemia in a large population-based study." *Clinical endocrinology* (2015).

81. Costantini, Antonio, and Maria Immacolata Pala. "Thiamine and Hashimoto's Thyroiditis: A Report of Three Cases." *The Journal of Alternative and Complementary Medicine* 20, no. 3 (2014): 208-211.

82. Thakur, Kiran, Sudhir Kumar Tomar, Ashish Kumar Singh, Surajit Mandal, and Sumit Arora. "Riboflavin and health: A review of recent human research." *Critical reviews in food science and nutrition* just-accepted (2016): 00-00.

83. Axe, Josh. "Vitamin B2/Riboflavin: Benefits, Sources, and Deficiency." https://draxe.com/vitamin-b2/ (Accessed October 3, 2016).

84. Cimino, Joseph A., Sunil Jhangiani, Ernest Schwartz, and Jack M. Cooperman. "Riboflavin metabolism in the hypothyroid human adult." *Proceedings of the Society for Experimental Biology and Medicine* 184, no. 2 (1987): 151-153.

85. Namazi, Nazli, Javad Heshmati, and Ali Tarighat-Esfanjani. "Supplementation with Riboflavin (Vitamin B." *Int. J. Vitam. Nutr. Res* 85, no. 1-2 (2015): 79-87.

86. Axe, Josh. Vitamin B5 / Pantothenic Acid Deficiency and How to Get Enough!" https://draxe.com/vitamin-b5/ (Accessed October 4, 2016).

87. Axe, Josh. "Vitamin B6 Benefits, Deficiency and Sources." https://draxe.com/vitamin-b6-benefits/ (Accessed October 4, 2016).

88. Axe, Josh. "Biotin benefits: Thicken Hair, Nails and Beautify Skin." https://draxe.com/biotin-benefits/ (Accessed October 4, 2016).

89. Kummer, Sebastian, Derik Hermsen, and Felix Distelmaier. "Biotin treatment mimicking Graves' disease." *New England Journal of Medicine* 375, no. 7 (2016): 704-706.

90. Barbesino, Giuseppe. "Misdiagnosis of Graves' disease with apparent severe hyperthyroidism in a patient taking biotin megadoses." *Thyroid* 26, no. 6 (2016): 860-863.

91. Cole, Bernard F., John A. Baron, Robert S. Sandler, Robert W. Haile, Dennis J. Ahnen, Robert S. Bresalier, Gail McKeown-Eyssen et al. "Folic acid for the prevention of colorectal adenomas: a randomized clinical trial." *Jama* 297, no. 21 (2007): 2351-2359.

92. Axe, Josh. "Folate vs Folic Acid...1 is Healthy and 1 is Dangerous." https://draxe.com/folate-vs-folic-acid-1-healthy-1-dangerous/ (Accessed October 5, 2016).

93. Ziaee, Amir, Nader Hajibagher Tehrani, Zahra Hosseinkhani, Amir Kazemifar, Amir Javadi, and Toktam Karimzadeh. "Effects of folic acid plus levothyroxine on serum homocysteine level in hypothyroidism." *Caspian journal of internal medicine* 3, no. 2 (2012): 417.

94. Shipton, Michael J., and Jecko Thachil. "Vitamin B12 deficiency–A 21st century perspective." *Clinical Medicine* 15, no. 2 (2015): 145-150.

95. Collins AB, Pawlak R. "Prevalence of vitamin B-12 deficiency among patients with thyroid dysfunction." *Asia Pac J Clin Nutr* 25 no. 2 (2016): 221-226.

96. Chan, Catherine Qiu Hua, Lian Leng Low, and Kheng Hock Lee. "Oral Vitamin B12 Replacement for the Treatment of Pernicious Anemia." *Frontiers in Medicine* 3 (2016).

97. Human Performance Resource Center. "Vitamin B Complex." http://hprc-online.org/dietary-supplements/files/monograph-vitamin-b-complex (Accessed October 8, 2016).

98. Osansky, Eric. "Vitamin A and thyroid health." http://www.naturalendocrinesolutions.com/articles/vitamin-a-thyroid-health/ (Accessed October 8, 2016).

99. Axe, Josh. "Vitamin A: Benefits, Sources and Side Effects." https://draxe.com/vitamin-a/ (Accessed October 6, 2016).

100. Farhangi, Mahdieh Abbasalizad, Seyyed Ali Keshavarz, Mohammadreza Eshraghian, Alireza Ostadrahimi, and Ali Akbar Saboor-Yaraghi. "The effect of vitamin A supplementation on thyroid function in premenopausal women." Journal of the American College of Nutrition 31, no. 4 (2012): 268-274.

101. Morley, John E., Robert M. Russell, A. Reed, E. A. Carney, and J. M. Hershman. "The interrelationship of thyroid hormones with vitamin A and zinc nutritional status in patients with chronic hepatic and gastrointestinal disorders." *The American journal of clinical nutrition* 34, no. 8 (1981): 1489-1495.

102. National Institutes of Health. "Vitamin A." https://ods.od.nih.gov/factsheets/VitaminA-HealthProfessional/ (Accessed October 7, 2016).

103. Enig, Mary and Fallon, Sally. "Vitamin A Saga." http://www.westonaprice.org/health-topics/abcs-of-nutrition/vitamin-a-saga/ (Accessed October 8, 2016).

104. Mackawy, Amal Mohammed Husein, Bushra Mohammed Al-Ayed, and Bashayer Mater Al-Rashidi. "Vitamin D deficiency and its association with thyroid disease." *International journal of health sciences* 7, no. 3 (2013): 267.

105. Kresser, Chris. "The Role of Vitamin D Deficiency in Thyroid Disorders." http://chriskresser.com/the-role-of-vitamin-d-deficiency-in-thyroid-disorders/ [Accessed October 11th, 2016].

106. Holick, Michael F., and Tai C. Chen. "Vitamin D deficiency: a worldwide problem with health consequences." *The American journal of clinical nutrition* 87, no. 4 (2008): 1080S-1086S.

107. Shukla, Kirtikar, Shikha Sharma, Aditi Gupta, Arun Raizada, and Kamini Vinayak. "Current Scenario of Prevalence of Vitamin D deficiency in Ostensibly Healthy Indian Population: A Hospital Based Retrospective Study." *Indian Journal of Clinical Biochemistry* 31, no. 4 (2016): 452-457.

108. Mackawy, Amal Mohammed Husein, Bushra Mohammed Al-Ayed, and Bashayer Mater Al-Rashidi. "Vitamin D deficiency and its association with thyroid disease." *International journal of health sciences* 7, no. 3 (2013): 267-275.

109. Kivity, Shaye, Nancy Agmon-Levin, Michael Zisappl, Yinon Shapira, Endre V. Nagy, Katalin Dankó, Zoltan Szekanecz, Pnina Langevitz, and Yehuda Shoenfeld. "Vitamin D and autoimmune thyroid diseases." *Cellular & molecular immunology* 8, no. 3 (2011): 243-247.

110. Vitamin D Council. "How do I get the vitamin D my body needs?" http://www.vitamindcouncil.org/about-vitamin-d/how-do-i-get-the-vitamin-d-my-body-needs/ (Accessed October 8, 2016).

111. Osansky, Eric. "Vitamin E and Thyroid Health." http://www.naturalendocrinesolutions.com/articles/vitamin-e-and-thyroid-health/ (Accessed October 8, 2016).

112. Patel, Viren, Cameron Rink, Gayle M. Gordillo, Savita Khanna, Urmila Gnyawali, Sashwati Roy, Bassel Shneker et al. "Oral tocotrienols are transported to human tissues and delay the progression of the model for end-stage liver disease score in patients." *The Journal of nutrition* 142, no. 3 (2012): 513-519.

113. Axe, Josh. "Vitamin E Benefits, Foods and Side Effects." https://draxe.com/vitamin-e-benefits/ (Accessed October 8, 2016).

114. Osansky, Eric. "Vitamin K and Thyroid Health." http://www.naturalendocrinesolutions.com/articles/vitamin-k-thyroid-health/ (Accessed October 8, 2016).

Lightning Source UK Ltd.
Milton Keynes UK
UKHW020621021219
354614UK00011B/1250/P